HEAI

This series introduces a wide range of healing techniques that can be used either independently or as a complement to traditional medical treatment. Most of the techniques included in the series can be learnt and practised alone, and each encourages a degree of self-reliance, offering the tools needed to achieve and maintain an optimum state of health.

Each title opens with information on the history and principles of the technique and goes on to offer practical and straightforward guidance on ways in which it can be applied, with diagrams and case studies where appropriate. Please note that readers are advised to seek professional guidance for serious ailments, and to make use of the list of practitioners for further guidance. Many of the techniques in this series are taught in workshops and adult education classes; all of the titles are written by professional practitioners with many years of experience and proven track records.

AVAILABLE IN THIS SERIES

Healing with Colour — Helen Graham

Healing with Crystals — Jacquie Burgess

Healing with Essential Oils — Nicola Naylor

Healing with Herbs — Judith Hoad

Healing with Homeopathy — Peter Chappell and
  David Andrews

Healing with Meditation — Doriel Hall

Healing with Osteopathy — Peta Sneddon and Paolo Coseschi

Healing with Reflexology — Rosalind Oxenford

Healing with Shiatsu — Catherine Sutton

FORTHCOMING TITLES IN THIS SERIES

Healing with Flower Essences

Healing with Nutritional Therapy

Healing with Ayurveda

ANGELA HOPE-MURRAY

TONY PICKUP

Gill & Macmillan

Gill & Macmillan Ltd
Goldenbridge
Dublin 8
with associated companies throughout the world
© Angela Hope-Murray and Tony Pickup 1997
0 7171 24568
Series editor: Tessa Strickland
Series copy editor: Pamela Dix
Index compiled by Helen Litton
Print origination by Carole Lynch
Printed by ColourBooks Ltd, Dublin
Original text design by Identikit Design Consultants, Dublin

This book is typeset in 10/15 pt Bembo.

A catalogue record is available for this book from
the British Library.

1 3 5 4 2

Contents

Acknowledgements

With thanks to the teachers: Dr Vasant Lad and
Dr Robert Svoboda; for many hours of help: Laura Miles.

CHAPTER ONE

What is Ayurveda?

Ayurveda means 'the science of life'. An ancient Indian medical system, it is holistic in the fullest sense of the term, in that it gives priority to the involvement of the patient in his or her own well-being.

Ayurveda empowers you to take control of your own life and health, with the aim of preventing illness, as opposed only to treating disease once it has arisen. For example, if you have a headache, you will not only be recommended a treatment that can be swallowed, rubbed in, or inhaled, but also asked to look at the imbalance in your lifestyle, your environment, diet and mind that has given rise to the pain. Once the imbalance is identified, there are some traditional remedies that are frequently helpful in the short term, but in the long term you are enabled to live in such a way that the cause of the pain never returns.

PERFECTION

We all seek the peace associated with perfect health of mind, body and spirit and would love to achieve perfect bliss (if we can believe that that is possible). Life is like a set of scales: it is possible, by using the appropriate measure of each of life's ingredients, for perfect balance to be achieved and illness to disappear. This balance is an integration of body, mind and spirit, leading ultimately to perfect bliss.

THE ELEMENTS

Health may be defined as perfect balance between body, mind, spirit and the environment. The basic tenet of

Ayurveda is that the body is composed of the elements earth, air, fire, water and ether. Our bodies are made up of combinations of these elements, as is the food we eat or anything else we come into contact with. Intake of, or contact with, a particular element will tend to increase that element within ourselves; so, eating a chilli will cause a sensation of heat because it is a fiery food. This also applies to our thoughts and the effect that they have on our physical bodies: we are what we think. Everything entering the body — heat, thoughts and experiences as well as food — must be first digested or else it will be incorporated into the being in a form which is unsuitable and will cause disease. Similarly, excesses or deficiencies in our diet, environment or thoughts, which the digestive process cannot compensate for, lead to excesses or deficiencies of particular elements in the body, creating imbalance and hence disease.

IMBALANCE AND ILLNESS

The aim of Ayurveda is to avoid excesses in life (food or otherwise) and to supplement what is deficient. Importantly, what may be sufficient for one person may be deficient or excessive for another, depending upon his or her basic constitution. All diseases are seen as caused by imbalance and thus can be resolved by paying attention to achieving balance whatever the patient is suffering from, be it a headache, depression, anxiety, insomnia, arthritis or asthma. As well as restoring balance, it is important that the actual cause of the imbalance is removed on an ongoing basis by appropriate attention to diet and lifestyle. There are some herbs which can help to create balance or to restore correct functioning in the alimentary canal for example, where food digestion takes place. The healthy intestine also regulates what is absorbed from the food we eat and is thus effective in maintaining balance.

In this book, we shall describe the various elemental forces acting in the body and mind and how they give rise to imbalance and illness. We shall also explain how they can function together in health. This book will empower you to change your life for the better and remove those annoying ailments we all tend to put up with. If you are thinking about visiting an ayurvedic practitioner, we shall tell you what to do before you go, what to expect once you get there and what it all means.

Today, the principles and practice of ayurvedic medicine are being increasingly employed by many, not only in India but also in Europe, Australasia and North America, as part of an holistic approach not just to disease, but to the entirety of everyday life.

CHAPTER TWO

The History of Ayurveda

The origin of Ayurveda can be traced to ancient times. The story in the *Charaka Samhita*, one of the oldest ayurvedic medical texts, runs like this. Fifty of the most eminent sages gathered together on the slopes of the Himalayas to discuss how to get rid of the common diseases which were causing so much ill health among human beings and interfering in the performance of their duties. They came to the conclusion that Indra, Lord of the Immortals, should be sought out, as he knew Ayurveda, or the science of life. This he was supposed to have learned from the physicians of the gods. They, in turn, had learned their knowledge from Brahma, the Creator. Sage Bharadvaya volunteered to go to Indra, who shared his knowledge. It proved most effective.

Many other versions abound, and are similar to stories in other cultures; just as Brahma explained Ayurveda to the Indians, so did Apollo and Thoth reveal the Greek and Egyptian systems of medicine to their respective peoples.

THE ORIGINS OF AYURVEDA

Let us now look at the 'facts' as far as they are known. It is difficult to be precise about the start of civilisation in India and about the historical origins of Ayurveda, as all dates are unrecorded prior to the time of Buddha (563-483 B.C.). The earliest civilisations appear to have been the Harappa, which existed in the Indus Valley, from *circa* 3000 B.C. until 1500 B.C. They were a successful race and achieved a society similar to that created in Rome much later. There is very little evidence of a medical system, although one must have existed. It was probably the Aryans, a group of people from the Caucasus, invading and mixing their systems with those of the Harappa, who introduced Ayurveda.

The Aryans brought with them a new body of wisdom and religious practice and probably took on some of the local Harappan customs. The books which record this knowledge, the *Vedas,* were probably first written around the time of this invasion; Ayurveda probably developed from the book known as the *Atharva Veda.*

Around 1000 B.C., knowledge in the classical texts of Ayurveda was further refined, giving rise to two textbooks, the *Charaka Samhita* and, much later, the *Sushruta Samhita.* This knowledge was further systematised in the Pauranic period (seventh century B.C.), when a text was produced on *Swastha-Vritta* or 'Regimen for Health'. This deals with *dinacharya* (daily routine) and *ritucharya* (seasonal adaptation). There is also a text known as the *Atur-Vritta* — 'Regimen in Disease' — in which over 1,000 diseases are described.

BUDDHISM AND AYURVEDA

Next came the Buddhist period, when knowledge of Ayurveda improved greatly. This was a golden age for this part of Asia and even in the sixth century B.C. a 'university', which became a centre of medical science, existed at Taxila near Rawalpindi. There is a story about one of the students, Jivaka, who was dispatched by his teacher to go and find a plant that could not be used as a medicine. He was unable to do so, and was later appointed by King Bimbisara as his royal physician and to be responsible for the well-being of the Buddha and his disciples. The royal physician was very important for

the stability of the 'state' and thus highly respected. His
endorsement by both the king and the Buddha ensured
his success — people came from far and wide to be
disciples of the Buddha just in order to be treated by him.

Although the Greeks were probably aware of Indian
culture and their medical systems, the invasion of
Northern India by Alexander the Great in 326 B.C.
was likely to have been responsible for the spread of
Ayurveda into Europe. Once again, endorsement was
the key factor; Alexander believed the system to be
very effective. Meanwhile, in northern India, an emperor
called Ashoka was also at work disseminating the
ayurvedic system. He established a local network of
hospitals and was very active in foreign relations, sending
envoys to bordering countries carrying with them news
of Ayurveda. A book on diagnostics appeared in the eighth
century and the Buddhist movement set up universities
to teach Buddhism, the wisdom recorded in the vedas and
other subjects, including medicine. One of these, Nalanda
university, thrived until about the twelfth century.

THE END OF THE GOLDEN AGE

This golden age came to an end when northern India
was invaded again. The invaders destroyed the universities
and burned the libraries. Some Buddhist monks escaped
to Tibet and as a result a number of ayurvedic texts are
preserved now only in a Tibetan translation. Nonetheless,
Ayurveda survived as a system of medical practice, and
documentation was maintained and added to as the
centuries passed. In the medieval period, sometime
between the twelfth and fifteenth centuries, in a new
textbook, the *Sarangakhara Samhita*, pulse examination
and its relation to the diagnosis of diseases is mentioned

for the first time. Then, during the sixteenth century, Akbar the Mogul emperor organised the unification of all Indian medical systems.

Indian spices had been highly treasured in Europe for many centuries, and as trade routes opened up during the sixteenth and seventeenth centuries Europeans developed a fashion for anything Indian. During their colonial rule of India, the British used local ayurvedic medicines because of the expense and difficulty of importing western medicine. However, the edict in 1835 that only European knowledge should be taught, together with the production of the British Pharmacopoeia in 1858, caused many physicians to move away from the use of local drugs. Furthermore, the state no longer funded ayurvedic training and over the next century much knowledge and understanding were lost. Fortunately the textbooks survived, and European surgeons translated and brought into practice a technique described in the *Sushruta Samhita* to repair damage to the face. This technique fostered the discipline we now call plastic surgery.

AYURVEDA TODAY

Since Indian independence in 1947, Ayurveda has received recognition throughout India and is one of the six systems officially recognised by the country's government. Qualified ayurvedic physicians have been and are being registered as medical practitioners. A number of hospitals are already established in which patients are treated according to ayurvedic tenets, and practical lessons are given to students.

CHAPTER THREE

The Philosophy of Ayurveda

To understand Ayurveda, it is important to understand something about its philosophy. Ayurveda is based on the Indian *samkhya* philosophy of creation. *Samkhya* comes from two Sanskrit words: *sat*, meaning 'truth' and *khya*, meaning 'to know'.

SAMKHYA

A central theme of *samkhya* philosophy is that the one absolute truth is absolute consciousness, an idea very similar to modern views about the origin of our universe, in that absolute consciousness represents a singularity. In the beginning, there was only one single essence. There was at that time no 'existence' — there was no *thing* in the universe. Even the universe did not exist! The universe is considered to be an expression of that singularity. In *samkhya* philosophy, there is a basic belief that the observable universe is only one of many manifestations of the absolute reality (in Sanskrit, *paramatma*). The *paramatma* is not limited in any way. Everything else in the universe, which is an expression of that reality, is limited. This is because the universe is constructed of opposites such as light and dark, near and far, and so on — in other words, we exist in a dualistic universe rather than in a singularity. Words are dualistic and limited, and we use words to describe everything. However, because everything is a representation of the absolute, the truth exists already within all things including human beings; it simply has to be realised and brought forth. This truth includes the information required for healing. We have only to discover and realise it.

AYURVEDIC PHILOSOPHY

According to *samkhya* philosophy, the primary force which pervades the universe is consciousness; matter arises from consciousness, not vice versa. All of creation is present only to glorify the absolute reality or absolute self. It is our illusion that the universe is stable; as we all now know, it appears to be constantly expanding, and if there is enough matter in the universe, it will eventually slow down and collapse again to a singularity.

Samkhya philosophy also states that the universe will go on collapsing and re-expanding over and over again for ever. The universe is governed by a set of rules, of which the most important perhaps is that all 'things' come to pass, or put another way, everything is constantly changing regardless of the illusion of stability. It is only God, or the absolute reality, which is beyond change.

People are not excluded from this rule of change; our bodies are constantly changing, albeit apparently slowly, as are our minds and our beliefs, with every new experience or piece of information which comes our way. Our environment is also changing, but it is made up of the same chemical elements as our physical form; the energy within the universe is no different to that in our minds. The aim of Ayurveda is to make sure that there is internal harmony and that the internal, or 'small', is in complete harmony with the environment, or 'big', at every level.

It is said, in *samkha* philosophy, that until the 'singularity', or absolute consciousness, desires to experience itself, it remains a singularity. In addition, because desire is the causative agent which brought the universe into being, it pervades all things. It generates duality from unity. The Genesis story in the Bible tells

essentially the same story, in that God divided the heavens
from the earth and the light from the dark, and so on,
implying that originally they were as one.

PRAKRUTI

The primary aspect of the created universe is nature, or
prakruti in Sanskrit; it is the complicated web of the
manifested universe. It is this difference between absolute
reality and nature which gives rise to the feeling of
separateness, that 'I' am different from the person next
door or playing a different role than 'I' was yesterday.
This 'I' is known as the 'ego', or in Sanskrit the *ahamkara*.
The *ahamkara* 'I' represents the physical and chemical
components and processes of the body, as opposed to the
true 'I', the soul, or that part of a being which is an
unchangeable part of the truth of creation, known in
Sanskrit as the *Atman*.

THE GUNAS

Ahamkara or the biochemical and physical processes of the
body may be considered as composed of an in-built, all
encompassing order, or equilibrium. The energy that
creates this equilibrium has three qualities, known as
gunas. They are: *sattva* (sometimes translated as purity and
also as subjective consciousness); *tamas* (darkness, inertia);
and *rajas* (activity, passion, the process of change). In the
human being, *sattva* is the ability of the five senses to react
in the way they do; it is not the sense organs themselves or
the process of nervous impulses travelling to the brain, but
simply the *ability* of those sense organs to be able to sense
what is available to be sensed. *Tamas* represents all that has
form and inertia, or resistance to being moved. In the case
of the sense organs, *tamas* represents their physical

structure. *Rajas* is the kinetic energy that links together *tamas* and *sattva*; for example, it includes the movement of impulses from the sense organs to the brain.

According to *samkhya*, these three *gunas* are continually separating and uniting, and are present in varying proportions in everything that makes up the physical world. Together they create the first cosmic soundless sound, AUM (OM), which continually operates in this universe.

We shall look at each of the gunas in turn and explore how they contribute to the world we perceive.

SATTVA

The expression of the soul which is part of, and continuous with, absolute consciousness is determined by the state of health of the body; the soul itself remains pure and unaffected. It is only its expression in the outside world that is modified by health or illness. *Sattva* is the essence of what is needed to make you and I the way we are, or at least the way we are meant to be — pure consciousness and bliss.

RAJAS

Rajas represents action or movement. It is an expression of all transfers of energy from one state to another, of all living metabolic processes and of all our physical activities. It provides the link between *tamas* (matter or inertia) and *sattva* (the subjective consciousness); it connects subject with object. *Rajas* and *sattva* unite together to produce eleven sense and motor organs which are the functioning structure of the human body.

While *sattva* and *tamas* are fundamental, *rajas* is a linking power; there would be no 'experience' if the force

of *rajas* was not present to enable the expression of the
other two. It is the quality of this vital co-existent balance
that is the central tenet of Ayurveda.

TAMAS

Tamas is divided into five principle parts, which give form
to the five senses: sound, touch, form, taste and odour.
These in turn give form to the division of the elements
that make up the universe.
They are:

- ether
- air
- fire
- water
- earth

These are the elements of the environment and of ourselves.

THE FIVE ELEMENTS

earth has the character of *solidity*
water has the character of *liquidity*
air has the character of *gas*
fire has the character of *change/energy*
ether has the character of *space*

Ether is a difficult concept for us in the west to grasp. It is
hard to understand how the space in which other things
exist can have a physical form — there appears to be
nothing in it by definition. Yet space is a part of physical
creation. Remember that we used to believe the sun
rotated around the earth, but now appreciate that the
reverse is true. If the universe is expanding, what is it
expanding into, if not space? The answer is that more
space is created as the universe expands — it does not exist
outside the universe.

Imagine that you are at the North Pole painting concentric circles on the ice, standing on unpainted ice, outside your circles. Paint more circles and eventually you will arrive at the South Pole; you are now standing at the South Pole on the inside of your circles! Extend this concept to a golf ball and cover it with coats of paint. If you keep on doing this it will eventually reach almost the size of the universe. At this point, by analogy with the paint circles on the earth, you will find yourself painting on the inside.

In other words, space is a physical feature of the universe and does not exist outside it — it is finite. Modern physics theory predicts, but has not yet proven, that all matter is composed of identical elementary particles. If shown to be true, then the same theory predicts that space will also be composed of the same particles. Therefore space, at the finest level of discrimination, has a physical form. This physical concept of space is synonymous with what is known in Ayurveda as 'ether'.

In Ayurveda, a person is composed of these five elements, plus consciousness. Given that it is our nature to be pure consciousness and bliss, and that the expression of the soul or consciousness is affected by the state of health of our bodies, you would expect that devotion to well-being should be our primary objective. Unfortunately, it is so often the third or fourth objective in our daily lives.

Desire is said to have caused the universe to spring into existence, probably because of an imbalance in the original singularity. Desire is also the force which causes imbalance in the body and thus 'illness'; this is especially true of selfish desire (in Sanskrit, *raga*). One of the desires of modern man is to live as long as possible, but this

ignores the possibility of living well. Ayurveda is
concerned with living well, not necessarily with living
longer; if the latter is the result of living well, that is fine,
but it should not be a primary desire in itself. Given the
choice of another forty years of life wracked with pain or
twenty years of pure bliss, which would you choose?

Living well implies achieving balance within the body,
mind and spirit, preventing disease from arising rather than
attempting to cure it once it has arisen. It is a way of life
involving balance in diet, work, play and rest. Only by
applying the appropriate measure of each of these
ingredients, will internal and external harmony be
achieved. Ayurveda enables us to be aware of what we
need and of what we do not need, and so make informed
choices for ourselves as to how to live and remain healthy.

CHAPTER FOUR

How does Ayurveda Work?

In Ayurveda, health is defined as perfect balance between body, mind, spirit and the environment; ayurvedic techniques focus on achieving that balance. Balance is achieved by the correct 'measure' of all things, although there is a thin line between enough and too much. Our desires usually cause us to lose sight of the correct measure in a particular circumstance; the most common desires causing this problem are those such as lust, hatred, fear, envy, arrogance or greed. The loss of measure causes imbalance in our lives.

We do most things in our lives because of one desire or another, and not just desires such as lust; there are four other fundamental desires:

- to live to see another day, and ultimately as many days as possible
- to do that which we were born to do (whatever we may believe that to be — *dharma* in Sanskrit)
- to have enough resources, usually money *(artha* in Sanskrit) to perform our *dharma* or destiny
- to be happy (we imagine by achievement of the previous three — *sukha* in Sanskrit).

This set of needs has been redefined in modern times by Abraham Maslow and presented as a 'hierarchy of needs'.

Desire causes lack of measure, which results in imbalance of the body and mind and so leads to disease; if everything is in balance then health prevails. We all know happy people who appear to be well most of the time and, conversely, sad people who seem to be ill all the time. An important path towards happiness and good health is liberation from the mind, where all our desires arise. But sadly, the mind and its desires control our actions, rule our lives and cause imbalance.

However, we all as children learnt the truism 'too much of a good thing is bad for you' and most of us know to our cost (usually after too much rich food), how accurate this is. How do we balance the way we lead our lives by always applying measure to everything we do and how can we discover what that measure is?

THE DOSHAS

In control of the living processes of the mind and the body and responsible for achieving and maintaining balance are three principle 'energies', or doshas. The Sanskrit word *dosha* is the root of the Greek prefix *dys*, used in English words such as dysentery or dysfunction, meaning 'fault'. These three doshas are called *vata*, *pitta* and *kapha* and they are arranged as follows:

- *vata* — a combination of air and ether
- *pitta* — a combination of fire and water
- *kapha* — a combination of water and earth

The state of perfect health is bliss or total 'stillness', but the nature of life is one of action and movement. So how can this bliss be achieved when our bodies and minds are vitalised by these three 'out of balance' forces? It is perhaps easiest to consider the state of body and mind as a triangle, with *vata*, *pitta* and *kapha* pulling or pushing at each of the three corners respectively. If the three forces are in balance, the triangle will remain perfectly still, whereas if one or more of them are out of balance with the others, then the triangle will move in the direction of the forces pulling the strongest. In both the body and the mind, this loss of stability, or disharmony, causes disease. The doshas each have specific activities in the body. *Vata* is responsible for motion in both the body and the mind. *Pitta* is in charge of any form of change. *Kapha* produces lubrication as well as insulation.

GENERAL FUNCTIONS OF THE THREE DOSHAS

Vata	Pitta	Kapha
transmission of nerve impulses	digestion of food	mucus in the gut to lubricate food movement
	metabolism	
circulation of blood through the heart and body	production of body heat	mucus in the airways to ease respiration and trap dust particles
breathing	discrimination	
	vision	synovial fluid to lubricate the joints
transport of secretions from all the glands	colour of skin and eyes	
		physical matter in the body
movement of food through the gut	production of hunger and thirst	insulation
excretion of urine and faeces	conversion of sensation into nerve impulses	staying power
		sleep
childbirth	thought processes	
		long-term memory
expression of emotion	appreciation	
	reasoning	flexibility of tissues
vitality	intelligence	
creativity		compassion
	confidence	
enthusiasm		patience stability

All bodies are made up of combinations of these elements and their resultant forces, as is our food or anything else we come into contact with.

When we are in balance, the five elements function together healthily; when they are out of balance and the 'triangle' is biased in one direction or another, the body appears to function abnormally and we become ill. It is important to understand that the doshas, while essential for the vital force of life, are themselves 'faults'. There is more than one level of balance. It is not sufficient, in the event of imbalance due to an excess of one *dosha,* to increase the other two believing that equilibrium will be restored. What is necessary is to decrease the influence of the one that is in excess.

Kapha

Kapha is largely occupied in the manufacture of the slippery, oily, thick, tenacious substances. These lubricating protective and adhesive compounds are essential to untroubled daily life; they ease the movements of one surface over another without friction and prevent entry of harmful bacteria and dust to the body. If *kapha* is inadequately cleared from the body or if there is an excess intake, an excess of these materials, such as mucus, develops. If this excess is not cleared, it leads to disease or increased susceptibility to disease, such as sinusitis. Insufficient *kapha* intake will result in dryness, not due to an excess of air but rather to inadequate lubrication resulting in roughness, discomfort and instability. Some forms of arthritis are the result of *kapha* disorders.

Pitta

Pitta is concerned with digestion and is responsible for the
production of stomach acid and biliary secretions vital to
the breakdown of food. Bile is, however, always excreted
ultimately along with the remainder of digestive waste
products via the faeces. In the event of obstruction or
slower than normal excretion of the faeces, the bile is
reabsorbed and creates a 'hot' condition in the body, or
inflammation. Excessive production of *pitta* creates excess
acid and bile, associated with burning sensations in the gut
and, in the mind, with a bilious nature. Inadequate
intake/production of *pitta* results in so-called 'cold'
diseases — a lack of energy and confidence.

Vata

One of the end products of *vata* is gas in the body, but it
is more significantly the motive force behind all
transmission of nervous impulses both in the brain and
the peripheral nerves. Excessive nervous activity is seen as
over-sensitivity and we often refer in a derogatory manner
to people with excess *vata* in the brain, as 'air-heads' or
'spaced out'. The expression of emotions may be
inappropriate and the heart rate unsuited to the needs of
the circulation. Someone with too much *vata* we would
term as 'being of a nervous disposition'. It cannot be a
comfortable way to exist.

The doshas are not in themselves entities such as enzymes,
air or mucus. They are simply forces pulling on the
corners of the triangle. They are rather like high and low
pressure zones in the atmosphere; apart from the weather
forecasters' map, we cannot see the different pressures, but
we do feel the winds that they cause and see things

moving in the breeze. The doshas have principle locations in the body: *Kapha* is located mainly above the diaphragm; *vata* below the navel, especially in the colon and bladder; and *pitta* lies in between these two in the region of the liver. Each of the three forces also predominate in specific organs, sometimes just one and sometimes two are in the majority. Although it is only in the body and mind overall that balance exists, each individual tissue expresses a variation in representation of the doshas which is suited to the nature of that tissue and represents 'balance' for that organ.

PREDOMINANCE OF THE DOSHAS

Vata	Pitta	Kapha
nerves	brain	brain
brain	liver	joints
spinal cord	spleen	mouth
heart	small intestine	head
ears	endocrine glands	neck
skin	skin	stomach
lungs	eyes	lymph
bones	blood	lungs
	sweat	heart
		oesophagus
		fat

The three doshas are further divided into five categories each, by reference to their specific functions.

FUNCTIONS OF THE DOSHAS

Kapha	*Pitta*
stomach mucus (*kledak*)	digestive juices (*pachaka*)
pleural and pericardial fluid (*avalambak*)	haemoglobin (*ranjak*)
	melanin (*bhrajak*)
saliva (*bodhak*)	rhodopsin (*alochak*)
synovial fluid (*sleshak*)	neurotransmitters (*sadhak*)
cerebrospinal fluid (*tarpak*)	

Vata, being the power behind all things moving, is classified in a slightly different way. Firstly, *prana vata*, being a forward moving force, is situated between the diaphragm and the throat; *udana vata* is positioned between throat and head and termed upward moving; *samana vata*, an 'equalising' air, exists between the diaphragm and the navel; *apana vata* is downward moving and in the lower abdomen; lastly, *vyana vata* pervades everything and is distributed throughout the core of the body.

THE LIVING PROCESS AND THE ENVIRONMENT

Everything entering the body — heat, light, sound, thoughts, experiences and food, must be first digested by the application of 'fire'(*agni* in Sanskrit), otherwise it will end up in a form which is unsuitable and will cause disease. For example, the digestion normally breaks down all proteins into small fragments which can safely be

absorbed. The poisonous nature of some deadly
mushrooms is due to the fact that some proteins from
them are very unusual and the digestive process is unable
to break them down properly. As a result, they are
absorbed undigested, and the presence of these foreign
proteins in the body causes a severe reaction — if
properly broken down, they would be nutritious rather
than deadly. If everything is correctly 'digested', the
doshas remain in balance. But if there is inadequate
digestion (a weak or faulty *agni*), then an imbalance in
the doshas is caused and disease will follow. This is
another part of the vicious circle, for an imbalance in the
doshas tends to cause weak or faulty *agni*. The effects of
individual doshas on the nature of this digestive fire,
which applies as much to the music we listen to as the
food we eat, is as follows:

- increased *vata* makes the digestive fire behave
  erratically, just like a wind blowing on a bonfire —
  one is never sure which way it will blow next and it
  can become unpredictable and dangerous
- increased *pitta* makes the fire fiercer, just like
  throwing petrol on a bonfire — the fire becomes
  much hotter, larger and all consuming
- increased *kapha* dulls the fire — just like throwing
  water or earth on a bonfire; the flames die down
  and it looks as though it may go out any moment; it
  may also take a long time to recover.

WASTE DISPOSAL MECHANISM

The doshas also affect every other process in the body, and
for the ayurvedic physician the next most important
system is the primary waste disposal mechanism — the
lower bowel and the production of faeces. All the

processes in the large bowel, including excretion, are very important to our health.

Disturbances of this function inevitably give rise to problems elsewhere. Increased *vata* here causes, as one might expect, erratic bowel movements ranging from constipation to diarrhoea. Increased *pitta* causes bowel motions to be soft and loose, but without the frequency or explosive nature of diarrhoea. *Kapha* excess has very little adverse effect here.

THE INDIVIDUAL CONSTITUTION

Every person is created different from the next — we all have our individual constitutions. Our unique characteristics are said to be generated at the moment of conception and relate to the constitutions of each parent, their thoughts and emotional attitude (*bhawana* in Sanskrit), the time of year and the environment. This basic fixed constitution with which we are born is called the *prakruti*. The dependence upon conditions at the time of conception is why parents are advised to avoid noxious substances such as alcohol and tobacco intake prior to the time of conception; this caution should also be extended to the state of mind and the environment at the time. This basic constitution expresses itself in the nature of people as follows.

Dosha:	Vata	Pitta	Kapha
Nature:	erratic	intense	laid back
Result:	unable to retain mass and dissipates energy	tendency to excess control of both energy and mass	retains mass easily with poor expression of energy

There are eight possible combinations of these doshas, making up the basic constitutional types:

Vata

Pitta

Kapha

Vata + Pitta

Pitta + Kapha

Kapha + Vata

Vata + Pitta + Kapha (unbalanced)

Vata + Pitta + Kapha (balanced)

The ideal constitution is when all three doshas are present and in balance; sadly, this is very unusual.

Conversely, the unbalanced *vata+ pitta+ kapha* constitution is almost always associated with constant health problems. The majority of us have a *prakruti* predominated by two doshas and a few have single *dosha* constitutions. Those with a dual *prakruti*, whilst not as prone to ill health as the out of balance tridoshic individuals, are nonetheless much more difficult to treat than those with a single doshic make-up. For them, disease may arise not only from each *dosha* individually but also from the combination of the two.

THE CURRENT (DAY-TO-DAY) CONSTITUTION (VIKRUTI)

The maintenance of balance is the primary goal of Ayurveda, the secondary goal being to bring back into balance what has gone 'out of whack' so that it may then be *kept* in balance. The current ratio of the doshas in the individual from day to day, known as the *vikruti*, is created by the food eaten, literature read, conversation, music, thoughts and so on. To achieve internal balance it is best if the *vikruti* is identical to the *prakruti*. The ayurvedic principle in this respect is that like increases like; thus a diet high in *pitta* will tend to increase the *pitta* imbalance in someone who has a *pitta prakruti* and conversely a diet low in *pitta* will tend to reduce the *pitta* factor in that person.

If we dive into a cold swimming pool or into the sea, the water temperature makes us feel cold eventually and will ultimately drop our body temperature. When we come out we shiver, creating a marked rise in metabolic activity (*pitta*), increasing again the heat within ourselves. Alternatively, we may go into a sauna and heat flows into our bodies, raising the temperature towards normal. Perhaps more importantly, in the sauna we 'feel' hot in the same way that we 'feel' cold under a cold shower. The child with a raging temperature is sponged with tepid water by its mother to bring the temperature down to a safe level. Thought also affects the functioning of the body; anger, anxiety and frustration are often associated with stomach ulcers and the pain from them, and vice versa. Pain does not have the effect of making us feel happy; we feel emotions and process our thoughts very differently depending upon whether we feel hot, cold or comfortable. In short, everything has its effect upon everything else and because of that we can take steps to alter our *vikruti* if we wish.

We are what we think we are. We are what we eat. We are what we do. So we have it within our power to choose to be healthy and ultimately to experience peace and bliss. To do this, we need to explore in some detail the nature of the items we eat and our everyday experiences so that we can predict whether they will each tend to worsen or improve the imbalance we have; it is quite rare

to find an individual whose *vikruti* is similar to their
prakruti. We all have to work at it consciously.

QUALITIES OF MATTER

In Ayurveda, there are ten basic pairs of qualities which
describe the nature of *all* things — actions, substances,
time and space:

 1 Heavy / light
 2 Dull / intense
 3 Hot / cold
 4 Oily / dry
 5 Smooth / rough
 6 Soft / hard
 7 Stable / mobile
 8 Subtle / gross
 9 Solid / liquid
10 Clear / sticky

The most significant of these qualities are hot/cold,
heavy/light and oily/dry.

Both the quality of a food and the strength of our
digestion determine the effect of any of these upon
our *dosha* balance. Their effect is also related to our
current state, or *vikruti*. Coming into a warm house
from cold weather outside gives us the impression that
the house is hot, whereas coming into a house at exactly
the same temperature when it is baking hot outside elicits
the response that the house feels pleasantly cool. In the
same way, people with different constitutions (*prakruti*)
respond very differently when placed in the same
environment. This is why some of us 'feel the cold'
more than others.

DIGESTION

Food, or any other 'input' for that matter, has to be digested. The results of food digestion are substances known in Sanskrit as *dhatus*, which are used to build the tissues of the body.

In Ayurveda, there is a sequence to the production of various elements that compose the body, with sundry waste products being produced along the way. The nutritional essence from the digested food is used to produce the first *dhatu*; the nutritional essence from that *dhatu* is transformed to produce the next *dhatu* in the sequence and so on. This is seen as a continual process of refinement, in that the 'essence' is refined each time. At each step of refinement, waste products are produced and these are expelled in one form or another from the body.

Nutrition begins when the first elements of 'essence' are extracted from the food by the digestive processes in the gut and become something referred to as *rasa,* meaning 'anything nourishing'. This extraction into *rasa* is slightly different from what we in the west understand by digestion; it applies not only to the physical/chemical components of the food but also to its appearance, taste, texture, colour and odour. The same is true for all experience, in that everything with which we have an interaction has these qualities, even though they may not have a biochemical structure that can be eaten. The colour of the room in which you are sitting or the clothes you are wearing at this moment, the sounds you can hear, the fragrances in the air, the words you are reading, the movement of air and the sensations of touch are all affecting your mind and body and are being converted into the *dhatus* of the body at every moment.

Modern intensive care units in hospitals play music to patients in persistent coma because they appear to recover more rapidly than in silence. The latest research has discovered that the playing of Baroque music at low volume increases the ability of the mind to learn and remember what it is reading about at the time the music is playing. It seems that the patterns in Baroque music are very similar to activity in those parts of the brain responsible for retention and recall; the external patterns are 'nourishing' and reinforce the patterns in the brain. In other words, similar qualities have a reinforcing effect on one another. This is in accordance with Ayurveda's principle tenet that like increases like and conversely that dislike causes reduction.

We have control over everything in our realm of experience if we choose to. However, the easiest to control and perhaps the most significant influence on our experience of the external environment is food. If you live in a climate that is not suited to your constitution or *prakruti*, there may be little that can be done to change it apart from emigrating, an option not open to most people. However, we can adjust what we eat to offset the adverse effect of the climate or environmental factors that cannot be controlled.

THE QUALITIES OF FOOD

Food has three main qualities — its taste, its strength and its effect. Of these, taste is extremely important because it has a marked effect upon the *rasa* produced. So eating different tastes will affect the personality and the health of the body regardless of the number of calories or amount of protein present. The body needs and indeed may actually crave certain tastes in order to achieve contentment and good health. There is a catch here, however, for there is a great tendency for us to be unable to separate the cravings of the body from those of the mind! The mind can be our friend but also our enemy. The mind can be the greatest craver of all and it usually craves for all the wrong things. The distinction between these two cravings is perhaps the most crucial step that we need to take in order to modify our health and well-being.

The tastes associated with food are: sweet, sour, salty, bitter, pungent and astringent. Pungent means sharp, burning or strong in food terms (caustic when referring to speech). Astringent is derived from the Latin *ad* plus *stringere*, meaning 'to draw tight'; it is akin to the sensation experienced when eating unripe bananas or pomegranate — they cause the mouth to pucker (in speech, the descriptive terms 'stern' or 'austere' are probably more appropriate). These tastes have different effects upon the doshas as follows:

- decreasing *vata*: sweet, sour, salty
- decreasing *pitta*: sweet, bitter, astringent (if *pitta* increased)
- decreasing *kapha*: pungent, bitter, astringent (if *kapha* increased)
- increasing *vata*: pungent, astringent, bitter (in excess)
- increasing *pitta*: sour, salty, pungent
- increasing *kapha*: sweet, sour, salty

The strength of something is related to its 'taste', but not necessarily that perceived as a sensation upon the tongue. 'Sweet' foods are more strengthening than sour foods, in the same way as beautiful art, music or words are 'stronger' than discordant music or art. The hierarchical order of strengths of the various tastes are sweet, sour, salty, bitter, pungent and, weakest of all, astringent.

By taking into account all the properties of the foods we eat and the activities we perform, it is possible to adjust them so that there will be an effect upon the *vikruti*, or our current constitution.

Lack of attention to these matters frequently leads to imbalance in the doshas, and as a result the digestive and metabolic fire (*agni*) in the various parts of the body becomes disturbed. If this fire of life is disturbed, it will not function correctly; the result is the production of improperly digested food or incorrect metabolism, culminating in the creation of *ama*. *Ama* is undigested food or a substance produced by inappropriate metabolism at any level — it is the cause of all disease. Imbalance in the mind due to emotional attachments also causes *ama*, which gives rise to mental disease. Mental imbalances can become physical ones and vice-versa.

The term 'imbalance' in the doshas means a difference of your current constitution from that which is your basic nature, or *prakruti*. This imbalance affects digestion and metabolism, but is of relatively little consequence until the *ama* produced begins to 'settle in' or affect a tissue of the body, usually one that already has a predisposing weakness. For a while, the tissue is relatively unaffected, but as time goes by the presence of increasing amounts of *ama* in the tissue leads to gross symptoms of disease. If these are allowed to go unheeded, then ultimately the *ama* 'overflows' from this tissue and you begin to experience symptoms in other tissues of the body, or in the mind.

Ama is considered to be the principle cause of disease, though illness can arise in other ways. For example, a considerable excess of *kapha* in the body can act to block the movement of *vata*. Movement of one sort or another is, as we all know, vital for the processes in the body and when it is 'blocked' it often gives rise to pain.

The theory of the causation of disease in the ayurvedic system is simple and straightforward, but in practice it can be extremely complex. For this reason, it is advisable to consult an ayurvedic physician to obtain an accurate and early diagnosis. The physician will be able to detect imbalances in the doshas of which you are perhaps not yet aware and, by re-balancing them, prevent disease that would have occurred in the future. The physician will also be able to distinguish disease and the symptoms caused by accumulation of *ama* from those caused by severe doshic imbalance. There are, however, many things you can do yourself to balance the doshas and so prevent, or even cure, disease.

CHAPTER FIVE

A Personal Step-by-Step Guide

The first thing to do in order to decide upon the most appropriate life style for yourself, is to determine, as accurately as possible, your *prakruti*, or basic constitution. There are many ways to accomplish this and it is probably best to use all of them and come out with an overall decision rather than opt for one or two things which may miss the whole picture. Read the descriptions below and answer the questions that follow each section honestly. Do not be tempted to choose a characteristic because it appears to 'fit in' with others or because you see one as 'preferable' to another. This can be very difficult! It may be best to ask a friend to complete the questions for you. If there is a question which you cannot answer, leave it blank.

BODY FRAME

People with a *vata* constitution are often very tall or very short. They are usually thin and somewhat gawky, have a small body frame with narrow shoulders and hips and have 'delicate' wrists and ankles. They are rather delicate, with limbs that seem too thin for their length and they frequently benefit from thin, tapering fingers. There may be disproportion in the body make-up, such that some parts seem light and others heavy. It is the nature of *vata* to be unpredictable, as discussed earlier. Owing to a lack of fatty tissues, particularly just under the skin, the wrists, knees, ankles and elbows may seem to stick out or be knobbly. Joints such as knees or elbows often 'click' when straightening. Any unusual bony features are usually indicative of the influence of *vata*. The absence of subcutaneous fat means that veins and tendons are also plainly visible. If you have many of these characteristics there is a strong *vata* element in you.

If you have a medium frame with average shoulders and hips, there is a strong *pitta* element in your constitution. Fingers and toes are neither skinny nor podgy and are of average length. Everything is in proportion and naturally slightly athletic.

Kapha predominant people have a medium to large frame with large bones, broad shoulders and wide hips. *Kapha* qualities are water and earth, stability and reserve, so it is not surprising that these people tend to be large and bulky. The back rows of the scrum in rugby are classically composed of this type of individual. The body proportions are in balance and all on the large side, the bones do not stick out, nor are the joints visible. The fingers and toes are often quite short and plump, the neck robust.

Please tick the features below which most describe you. Key features are marked with a #.

Characteristic	*Vata*	*Pitta*	*Kapha*
Size at Birth #	❑ Small	❑ Medium	❑ Large
Height #	❑ Exceptionally short or tall	❑ Average	❑ Short and stocky; tall and large
Anatomical Features #	❑ Bony joints that crack, prominent veins	❑ Well proportioned	❑ Broad shoulders, strong muscles

WEIGHT

Vata types are usually thin. These are the people who eat
vast amounts of food, go back for seconds and have
pudding as well, yet never seem to put on one gram in
weight! Everyone else envies them, but seldom
understands that the *vata* person is actually trying to put
on a little weight, and is extremely frustrated because he
cannot, however much he tries. All the energy from the
food is spent in nervous energy and movement both inside
and outside the body, so there is nothing left for storage as
fat. *Vata* types are often referred to as 'skin and bones'.
One of the reasons they stay this way is because their diet
is often fairly balanced regardless of quantity; however, the
desire to gain weight can lead to eating a diet designed just
for weight gain and unbalanced. In this way, it is possible
for some of these people to become overweight, and
almost certainly ill at the same time. If a good diet is
resumed, they can quite easily lose the excess weight and
recover an overall sense of well-being.

   Pitta people find it easy to keep their weight steady
and are usually in the middle of the 'ideal weight for
height' tables. They do not develop midriff bulges if they
put on weight, but tend to distribute the weight evenly
over the body. *Pitta* is the fire/metabolism/balance force in
the constitution and so they can put on weight if they
wish to, or lose it by increasing exercise if required.

   On the other hand, those with a *kapha* constitution
need to exercise if they are to keep their weight to a
reasonable level. They are generally heavier for a given
height than the other two classes. These are the people
who can gain weight 'just by looking at a bowl of soup'.
They find it difficult to lose the weight they have put on
over the years, very often on the buttocks and legs. It is

their nature to store energy as fat and be 'heavy'. Ultimately, if the process is allowed to continue, the deposition of fat will begin to involve the other areas of the body as well. When the time comes to lose weight, they find that it disappears from the top half of the torso, then the waist, but seems to be almost impossible to lose around the buttocks and legs.

Please tick the feature below which *most* describes you.

Characteristic	Vata	Pitta	Kapha
Weight	❏ Light, hard to gain weight	❏ Moderate, gains and loses weight easily	❏ Heavy, difficulty losing weight

HAIR

To some extent, as with skin colour, the nature of your head hair is related to your racial background. Some races in northern Europe, or in the Far East especially, have typically straight hair, whereas inhabitants of the African continent tend towards the distinctly curly. So it is important to assess your hair as similar, straighter or curlier than one might anticipate given the average nature of hair in your racial group.

Vata people have dry hair on their heads more often than not but, as with the skin, it may be variable across the scalp. It is seldom naturally blond and tends to have a coarse or rough texture. It is usually quite curly and occasionally frizzy or tightly kinked. Dandruff is common. Because the hair also lacks emollients to keep it supple and shiny, the *vata* individual suffers split ends and dry, lacklustre hair. Body hair is either sparse or in excess — dark, rough and curly.

Pitta is the fire principle and fire is red, so if you have naturally red hair *pitta* features strongly in your *prakruti*. If *pitta* people are not red haired, they have blond or light brown hair, or their hair goes grey or white as early as their twenties. Premature hair loss in men is also a feature of strong *pitta*. The hair is usually thin and fine, quite straight and almost impossible to style without the use of hair gel or body enhancers. The high output of oils by the *pitta* skin on the scalp can result in the hair being so oily that it appears flat; in addition, dust may stick readily to this excess oil and cause dullness. Body hair is also white to light brown in colour and very fine.

Hair that is brown to dark brown, thick and slightly wavy rather than really curly (see *vata* hair above) is characteristic of the *kapha* influence. There is usually a moderate amount of body hair.

Please tick the features below which *most* describe you.

Characteristic	*Vata*	*Pitta*	*Kapha*
Hair colour (relative)#	❑Very dark	❑Fair/red/ light brown	❑Medium brown
Hair thickness#	❑Medium	❑Fine	❑Thick
Texture#	❑Coarse	❑Silky	❑Soft
Form#	❑Curly	❑Straight	❑Wavy

NAILS

Hard, brittle nails which crack and split easily with ridges are suggestive of a *vata prakruti*. As ever, irregularity of size and structure is typical of *vata*. Nail biters and pencil chewers are usually *vata* types. The nails of a *pitta* person are soft, but strong and smooth. The nail bed tends to be reddish in colour. *Kapha* nails are strong, large, thick and regular. The thickness may cause the nail bed to appear pale.

Please tick the features below which *most* describe you.

Characteristic *Vata*		*Pitta*	*Kapha*
Nail colour	❏ Pale	❏ Red	❏ Opaque
Nail strength	❏ Brittle	❏ Strong	❏ Tough
Nail size	❏ Irregular and ridged	❏ Regular	❏ Regular/ almost square

EYES

Eye colour is not easily determined for some people; in answering the following questions, use the underlying eye colour and ignore any small spots or flecks. Also, remember that once again different races tend to have specific ranges of eye colour and your answers must be in relation to that range. Eye size is subjective, so you may wish to ask someone else to comment on the size of your eyes as well as how much they move normally.

Vata constitutional eyes are characteristically grey to grey blue in the iris (the circle around the black pupil) but can also be very dark brown; if you have eyes of different colours, then the variable influence of *vata* is at work again. *Vata* people's eyes are often 'dry' and it frequently feels as though there is something caught under the eyelid. They can seem somewhat dull and are usually a little small. They appear constantly on the move, darting from one side to the other apparently tirelessly, but are in fact consuming energy under the influence of *vata* that is thus not available to be converted into fat.

The eyes of the *pitta* person generally range from hazel through green to light blue, including iridescent blue.

They are medium in size and easily inflamed. Indeed, even
in health, there are usually one or two blood vessels visible
in the sclera (the white part around the iris). *Pitta* eyes
have a sharp steady gaze and can be quite penetrating,
seeming at times almost to have the power to burn a hole
in the object or person being observed. Large, moist, mid
brown/dark blue, olive shaped eyes are typical of the *kapha*
constitution. Neither is movement rapid nor the gaze
intense; these eyes seem to exude softness.

Please tick the features below which *most* describe you.

Characteristic	*Vata*	*Pitta*	*Kapha*
Eye colour (relative)	❑ Dark brown or different	❑ Hazel, green, light blue, intense	❑ Mid brown/ dark blue
Eye size*	❑ Small	❑ Medium	❑ Large
Eye movement*	❑ Rapid and incessant	❑ Sharp, steady	❑ Slow

You may wish to ask someone else's opinion on these.

SKIN

Your skin colour is determined largely by your parents'
racial background, but also by the nature of, and your
exposure to, the environment in which you live. A
northern European who seems well tanned will still be
very much lighter in skin tone than the palest person with
an African heritage. This is a relative subject, and you
need to compare your colour to the members of your
family and with others of your race in order to be
accurate. This may be a question which it is easier to ask
one of your parents or friends from your racial group. It is
not easy if your parents are from widely different racial
backgrounds, in which case it may be better not to answer
the question on colour.

The *vata* person is rather on the dark side compared with their compatriots; they tan easily and do not tend to burn. They love the sun and heat and are always seeking it; they get a buzz from being out in the sunlight. This is because *vata* is, by its very nature, cold; *vata* dominated people do not store much energy to keep warm, so they actually need the heat. Their skin appears cold to other people, and often has a greyish hue. They always, with reason, complain that their circulation is bad and they suffer interminably from cold feet.

Pitta people generally have light coloured skin, often pinkish. They have a ruddy glow and often are covered in freckles; tanning is difficult for them — they burn readily and can suffer from unpleasant allergic reactions to sunlight. They have naturally warm/hot skin as perceived by others. With *kapha* as your constitutional type you enjoy sunbathing, but can burn (though not as readily as *pitta* types). The skin is cool — though not as cold as the *vata* person's to the touch — but cold hands and feet are unusual.

Please tick the features below which *most* describe you.

Characteristic	Vata	Pitta	Kapha
Skin colour (relative)#	☐ Dark	☐ Fair	☐ 'White'
Skin temperature*	☐ Cool	☐ Hot	☐ Warm
Tendency to burn#	☐ Low	☐ High	☐ Moderate
Tanning ability	☐ Easy	☐ Poor	☐ Moderately easy

*Ask someone else to answer this one for you.

Skin Characteristics

Dry skin is the lot of the *vata* person. The constant
movement and high energy expenditure means that
the little moisture there is in the skin rapidly disappears.
Once again, the unpredictable nature of *vata* comes
into play and whilst some parts of the skin may be dry,
others may be normal; if *vata* is particularly strong,
the skin may be dry everywhere. A lack of lubricating,
emollient substances in the skin results in cracking,
peeling and, when exposed to the sun, a somewhat
leathery or wrinkled appearance (though not burnt).
Cold weather can, paradoxically, have a similar effect
on the *vata* skin — if you always have to apply additional
lubricants to your lips in the winter to prevent them
from drying out, then *vata* is in your primary
constitution.

Pitta people frequently have fine skin, are
somewhat prone to developing rashes and particularly
show a tendency to acne in adolescence, but also
throughout their lives. Moles are common and owing
to the potentially increased rate of internal metabolism,
the skin's elastic tissues develop problems earlier than
most people's, meaning wrinkles appear sooner. *Pitta*
people become flushed easily on exertion — they
actually look hot. As you might expect, blushing
comes almost as second nature to the *pitta*. Individuals
with a *kapha* constitution have somewhat oily, almost
waxy, smooth, thick skin with few wrinkles. It is well
supplied with emollients from the body's own sources.
The skin is almost too uniform in terms of texture;
this is not just because there is more subcutaneous fat
underneath it, but relates to *kapha's* stable nature —
the antithesis of *vata*.

Please tick the features below which *most* describe you.

Characteristic	*Vata*	*Pitta*	*Kapha*
Skin surface	❑ Dry, prone to chapping and psoriasis	❑ Fine, prone to acne and rashes	❑ Smooth and waxy
Wrinkles	❑ Fine, in sunlight	❑ Early	❑ Very few

SWEAT

Remember that this set of qualities and questions is aimed at your *prakruti*, or basic constitution, and not necessarily exactly how you are now; so it can be helpful to think back to when you were a child. If you have a marked imbalance now, resulting in an increase in weight and subcutaneous fat, then it may be that you have a tendency to sweat more than you used to. Try to answer this question by considering how you were in your childhood.

The *vata* person hardly sweats at all, even when the weather is hot. They seem to need to absorb heat and there is little activity in the sweat glands directed to reducing body temperature. The handshake is always dry and usually cool. The high metabolic rate in *pitta* people means they may have a need to lose excess body heat, to keep their temperature normal, even when the weather is cold. These are people who are always sweating; the handshake is slightly damp, though generally hot as well. For *kapha*, the tendency to sweat is average; the handshake may be slightly damp, though rather cooler than in the case of a *pitta* make up.

Please tick the feature below which *most* describes you.

Characteristic *Vata*	*Pitta*	*Kapha*
Sweat ❑ Little	❑ Much	❑ Moderate

MOUTH AND LIPS

In keeping with the nature of *vata*, the jaw is either
too small or too large, so the teeth do not fit in the
mouth evenly. There is often great variability in the
sizes of individual teeth and, like the nails, they are
rather brittle with thin enamel. There is an increased
sensitivity of the teeth to cold and hot. The tongue is
frequently thinly coated, but be careful, as the tongue
is easily affected by your current nature (*vikruti*) and
so just looking at it in a mirror may be misleading with
regard to your *prakruti*. The lips are thin, occasionally
almost non-existent.

Pitta mouths have regular jaws, even teeth of
medium size and they all fit together well. High
metabolic activity means cavities frequently occur in
these teeth unless they are kept scrupulously clean.
The gums are soft and reddish and the teeth tend to
be yellowish. The tongue is often coated but frequently
appears red and may even seem inflamed. The lips are
clearly defined and on the full-coloured, red side.
Lucky *kapha* individuals have large, evenly sized, strong
white teeth which are generally resistant to disease.
The tongue is seldom coated, but if it is, it tends to be
thick and white. Their lips are very full — fuller than
pitta lips though perhaps not so well defined — and
always moist.

Please tick the features below which *most* describe you.

Characteristic	*Vata*	*Pitta*	*Kapha*
Teeth	❑ Uneven/ crooked	❑ Regular/ off white	❑ Regular/ white
Lips	❑ Thin	❑ Well defined, of moderate thickness	❑ Full and moist

APPETITE

Vata individuals are always 'hungry', but as their eyes are often larger than their stomachs their appetite is soon satisfied. The appetite varies from day to day and from meal to meal, in accordance with the character of *vata*. These constitutions often 'need' to eat between meals to prevent tiredness or dizziness. People with *pitta* featuring strongly in their constitution have robust appetites and always enjoy eating. The desire for food is less variable than the *vata* person's and while there is less tendency to eat between meals, these people dislike missing meals or changing the time when they eat. *Kapha* people have regular appetites, usually moderate, though they may eat at times just to fill their time. They are able to fast without any great problem, as they have so much energy stored as fat.

Please tick the feature below which *most* describes you.

Characteristic	*Vata*	*Pitta*	*Kapha*
Appetite#	❑ Erratic, constantly eating, but soon 'full'	❑ Strong/ excessive, need regular meals	❑ Steady, can go without eating

THIRST

One day the *vata* type will be constantly thirsty and it may
seem that no matter how much he drinks his thirst cannot
be quenched. Much of this desire is, however, in the mind
and typically these are people who get a drink and then
find it later, half finished. *Pitta* people tend to be
excessively thirsty. They need to drink regularly and
become very thirsty if they miss a routine drink at a
particular time of the day. The *kapha* individual never
really feels thirsty, unless he is perspiring a lot. The mouth
is always moist and he leave drinks unconsumed, not so
much because the desire is in the mind more than the
body, but because he simply does not feel particularly
thirsty.

Please tick the feature below which *most* describes you.

Characteristic	Vata	Pitta	Kapha
Thirst	❑ Variable, lots of drinks half drunk	❑ Always drinking	❑ Low

BOWEL MOVEMENTS

In health, the bowels move once or twice a day without
the need of laxatives or hard effort. If your bowels do not
move once a day with occasional rare exceptions, then
you are suffering from constipation. If the bowels move
three or more times a day and the stool is loose, then
diarrhoea is present.

Many people believe that the passed stool is the
residue of food not digested and absorbed in the small
intestine; in health, this is not true. The stool consists
mainly of dead cells from the lining of the gut (they are
all totally replaced every couple of days), together with

dead bacteria from the large part of the gut (colon). These bacteria are extremely important to the health of the entire gut; they are critical for the digestion of certain food substances that enter the large bowel (mainly soluble fibre, not to be confused with insoluble fibre such as bran). They convert this special form of soluble fibre to substances that are essential for the nutrition of the tissues in the gut itself. They are the digestive fire of the large bowel. Like the cells of the lining of the gut, which turn over rapidly and therefore need constant nutrition to be recreated, they have a limited life and must be excreted regularly. Indeed, if a person fasts, the weight of the stool changes very little from when they are eating. If food particles are present in the stool, then the fire in either the large or the small bowel, or both, is probably inadequate.

Vata people frequently complain of constipation; the stools tend to be hard, dark and difficult to pass; they suffer often from wind and at times may become bloated or experience gurgling noises in the abdomen. In common with the other characteristics of *vata* types, they may experience variability, with spells of diarrhoea in between periods of constipation. The *vata* person knows that occasionally he has to use dietary adjustments to normalise his bowel habits, or even resort to strong laxatives. The *pitta* person is one whose bowel habits are as regular as clockwork. The stools are usually well formed, but can be loose at times and may cause a burning sensation following a spicy meal. Regular bowel movements once a day are characteristic of a *kapha* constitution. The stools are routinely well formed.

Please tick the feature below which *most* describes you.

Characteristic	*Vata*	*Pitta*	*Kapha*
Bowel movements#	❑ Gassy, erratic, hard and dry with bouts of constipation	❑ Regular, occasionally loose	❑ Heavy, bulky, often sinks

SEX DRIVE

The sex drive or libido of the *vata* person is extremely variable from day to day; it can be affected by fantasies and can appear to be 'all or nothing'. Excessive expenditure of effort in sexual intercourse leaves the *vata* person tired owing to a lack of stored energy. Strong, passionate sexual desire typifies the *pitta* personality. Passion is readily aroused and fulfilled if possible. The *pitta* person, frequently being the one to initiate intercourse, takes control of it. Being clear about what they want tends to mean they become upset if they do not achieve it. Once again, the *kapha* individual demonstrates stability, loyalty, staying power and balance. They are almost never as intense as the *pitta* type and are slow to become aroused; however, once stimulated, their sexual energy declines very slowly.

Please tick the feature below which *most* describes you.

Characteristic	*Vata*	*Pitta*	*Kapha*
Libido	❑ Variable — all or nothing	❑ Passionate, domineering	❑ Steady, loyal, slow but sustained

MENSTRUATION

Menstruation can be the most difficult aspect of body function to assess, because every woman's view of what is normal or heavy is coloured by her experience over the years. The *vata* woman may experience a period which is for her heavy, but which a *pitta* woman would regard as light. Women with a *vata* constitution frequently have very irregular cycles; they classically miss periods when exercising too much or eating insufficiently. Periods are often late, but can be early too. The flow is variable, sometimes scanty and sometimes causing clots. The flow is often dark in colour. Sometimes there is constipation and abdominal cramping pain a few days before the period actually starts. Women with a *pitta* constitution usually have reliably regular cycles, but the loss tends to be for five or six days and can be quite heavy. It is bright red and cramps can be quite troublesome. Women with a *kapha* constitution have regular periods, with relatively little experience of cramping, but do tend to be troubled by water retention manifested often by a marked feeling of fullness in the breasts.

Please tick the feature below which *most* describes you.

Characteristic	*Vata*	*Pitta*	*Kapha*
Menstruation	❑ Variable, scanty, erratic	❑ Regular, heavy with cramps	❑ Regular, with premenstrual water retention

PULSE

The pulse should preferably be tested first thing in the morning before breakfast. It is a very important part of ayurvedic diagnosis, first introduced in the thirteenth

century A.D. It is a complex and acquired skill to be able
to assess the balance of the doshas from the nature of the
pulse and is best performed by an ayurvedic physician. It is
possible to discern the *prakruti* and also the *vikruti,* but this
is an art that requires many years of patient practice. You
can, though, check certain aspects of your own pulse as
follows.

Sit quietly for five or ten minutes, away from any
sources of direct heat, and breathe quietly. Turn the
right hand palm upwards and wrap the second, third
and fourth fingers of the left hand under the right wrist
until they are resting on top of the wrist, just in line
with the second finger of that hand, two fingers' width
from the hand itself. Press gently with the finger tips
and you will be able to feel the radial pulse. Now
decrease the pressure of your fingers tips slightly and
take note of the characteristics of the throbbing beat
of the pulse. Your index or second finger denotes the
vata dosha, the middle finger the *pitta dosha* and the
ring finger the *kapha dosha.* The strongest pulse is the
dosha that is predominant in the body. The doshas are
also responsible for the nature of the pulse itself: *vata*
controls the rhythm/regularity, *pitta* determines the
speed and *kapha* the volume.

The *vata* pulse is thin and thready, often with a
rhythm that varies markedly as you breathe — it may
even be highly irregular. When *vata* predominates, the
pulse appears to move in waves like a snake. The pulse
of a purely *pitta* person is regular and strong, about
seventy beats per minute, and varies only slightly as you
breathe; it is said to 'jump' like a frog. A *kapha* pulse is
powerful, full, slow and regular; it is likened to the
swimming of a swan.

Please tick the features below which *most* describe you.

Characteristic	*Vata*	*Pitta*	*Kapha*
Strongest pulse under	❑ Index finger	❑ Middle finger	❑ Ring finger
Nature	❑ Feeble, irregular, 90 per minute	❑ Regular, prominent 70–80 per minute	❑ Full, steady, 60–70 per minute

SPEECH

Vata people are able to speak about almost anything. Often however, you may find yourself talking about something completely different from what you started off with. Your voice tends to be 'breathy' and you love speaking, especially with another *vata* person, for hours on end.

If *pitta* is your constitution, the precision and fire of your make up will come through in your voice. You know what you want to say and the sort of response you expect from the listener. Your tone may carry impatience in it and you will often feel impatient to say what you wish to communicate. Conversations with another *pitta* individual tend to develop into arguments, or at least heated discussions. You are someone who speaks your mind — often regardless of the consequences. Slow and measured speech is the hallmark of the *kapha* person. You think carefully about what you say and don't give too much away. You may be reticent to communicate. What you do say is important and is conveyed with weight, using a mellifluous tone of voice. When talking with another *kapha* person, there tend to be large gaps in the conversation, which cause no discomfort to either party. This contrasts with the *pitta* individual, who feels the opportunity has come to pour out what he has been burning to say; and with the *vata*, who feels he must fill the silence with anything, relevant or not.

Please tick the feature below which *most* describes you.

Characteristic	Vata	Pitta	Kapha
Speech	☐ Fast, high pitched, changing from one subject to another	☐ Intense, and incisive; loves debate	☐ Slow and measured, low pitched

PHYSICAL ACTIVITY

Vata people are very active and frequently restless; always on the move, they fidget constantly but with little staying power. Their appetite is driven to a large extent by their most recent physical activity; hard work makes them hungry. Their coordination is often poor and they are prone to sudden bursts of activity which achieve no particular purpose. Activities can be left uncompleted through lack of stamina. *Vata* people relish frequent hard exercise, because of addiction to the internal morphine-like substances (endorphins) released by the body in response to exertion.

Individuals with a *pitta* make up can sustain prolonged hard exercise, but it tends to make them feel rather hot. Such exercise increases their thirst as much as the appetite. These are competitive people who often love sports. A *kapha* constitution is exemplified by lethargy; they do not generally wish to exercise, although if they do, it does not affect the appetite, which tends to be constant. High energy expenditure causes sweating, though at a moderate pace it may seem they can go on

forever without difficulty; sudden bursts of extreme
energy are not their style.

Please tick the feature below which *most* describes you.

Characteristic	*Vata*	*Pitta*	*Kapha*
Activity	❏ Very active, tends to fidget, expends energy quickly with poor endurance	❏ Moderately active, generally has lots of energy — likes sports and has desire to win	❏ Lethargic, slow moving but with excellent stamina and coordination

SLEEP

Vata people wake from sleep easily and tend to sleep
restlessly. Their sleep patterns are, predictably, variable.
They often grind their teeth at night and not infrequently
sleep-talk; the mind is still active, even though they are
supposed to be resting. They awake in the morning often
feeling unrested. *Pitta* people fall asleep readily, sleep
lightly and wake up ready to take on the new day. If they
should wake up during the night they go back to sleep
without any difficulty. The *kapha* person rapidly falls into
slumber while reading or listening to music; they sleep
deeply and are seldom roused during the night. Sleep
comes easily at any time of day or night.

Please tick the feature below which *most* describes you.

Characteristic	*Vata*	*Pitta*	*Kapha*
Sleep	❏ Light, fitful, unrefreshing, sleep talking	❏ Easy, short, refreshing	❏ Heavy, prolonged, slow to wake

DREAMING

People with a *vata* constitution dream profusely, or at least
are aware of their dreams because they wake so frequently;
by the time morning comes however, they have forgotten
what the dreams were about. Dreams are usually filled
with activity. Motion is common, especially the sensation
of being able to fly. *Pitta* dreams are also intense,
frequently passionate, and can be remembered the next
day, at least for a while. *Pitta* dreams are frequently in
colour; particularly vivid colours can be recalled later,
with an intensity that is typical of the *pitta* constitution.
Kapha in the constitution causes emotional rather than
passionate dreams. Frequently they are calm, relaxed,
matter-of-fact dreams of situations rather than any
sensation of movement.

Please tick the feature below which *most* describes you.

Characteristic	Vata	Pitta	Kapha
Dreams#	❑ Filled with activity, easily forgotten	❑ Passionate, in colour, remembered	❑ Relaxed, emotional, not easily remembered

EMOTIONAL TEMPERAMENT

This aspect of your nature is related to how you react
when facing a difficult situation. This is how you feel
under these circumstances, not necessarily the emotional
response which you display; you may have been taught to
react in defined ways, but this seldom affects how you
actually feel. *Vata* people show fear and anxiety as a first
reaction to any potentially threatening situation outside
their control. If you are of this type, then you experience a
dry mouth and a degree of panic. Thoughts will fly

around your mind in a chaotic jumble. *Pitta* is fire, which tends to ignite passionate feelings such as anger or a clear response, knowing exactly what to do for the best. Your thoughts are ordered and logical and the response straightforward and precise.

If you are a *kapha* person, you stay away from stressful situations because you do not like change. This may be such a strong trait that you bury your head in the sand rather than face the circumstances. Sometimes the situation does go away, but if not, then your emotional response tends to build up inside and may seriously accumulate over time. This can result, paradoxically, in unexpected reactions occasionally.

Please tick the feature below which *most* describes you.

Characteristic	*Vata*	*Pitta*	*Kapha*
Emotion#	❏ Anxious, insecure and unpredictable	❏ Forceful, irritable and jealous	❏ Calm but attached

CREATIVITY

There is a constant movement of ideas in the mind of the *vata* individual and a readiness to connect the apparently unconnected leads to great creativity. New ideas springing from the old make these people excellent at coming up with new theories, which may be seen by some as 'crazy'. As for implementing or testing new ideas, their tendency to be changeable and inability to focus means this is best left to the other types.

Pitta characters are excellent at the first stage of implementing a new idea. They have the passion to make sure the idea works. Their creativity is in the realm of modifying an original idea so that it works in practice. Once they have achieved this goal though, they will then move on to the next idea. It is very much the 'doing' that is important to them. The organisation of a project or dealing with the day-to-day detail is best left to a *kapha* person.

Kaphas have both feet on the ground. They have the tenacity to polish something until it positively shines. This is equally creative, but at the opposite end of the spectrum from the *vata* type. Kaphas are brilliant organisers, although occasionally their determined nature can lead to inflexibility.

Please tick the feature below which *most* describes you.

Characteristic	Vata	Pitta	Kapha
Creativity	❑ New ideas, flashes of inspiration	❑ Practical, molding, developing ideas and making them work	❑ Polishing, refining, good at organising others

MEMORY

A short memory is characteristic of *vata* people. They seldom hold grudges — they simply can't remember long enough to be able to. What happened recently can be remembered extremely well, but remote memory is almost non-existent. The *pitta* memory is sharp — these people remember easily and do not readily forget. *Kapha* individuals find it difficult to remember something and need to hear or experience it more than once before it becomes fixed in the mind. However, 'once remembered, never forgotten' is the motto that applies.

Please tick the feature below which *most* describes you.

Characteristic	*Vata*	*Pitta*	*Kapha*
Memory	❑ Recent memory good, past memory poor	❑ Very sharp	❑ Slow to commit to memory, but never forgets

PERSONALITY

Vata people are highly susceptible to external influences and react quickly to changes in their circumstances. Change in all things at all times is typical; one minute they desire company and a moment later need solitude. It can be difficult to keep up with their changeable moods, one minute ecstatic, the next depressed. Friendships come and go. They seem unwilling to adopt any pattern in their daily existence, to the extent that they seldom finish what they start. If motivated, they can be the driving force behind anything, the life and soul of the party, but will seldom be there at the end. Many of their decisions and emotions arise from feelings of uncertainty.

Pragmatic, clear and powerful in their actions and emotions, *pitta* characters can become domineering. They are always passionate and thus intrinsically brave but well balanced. This passionate nature leads to reliable enthusiasm and commitment, but can be negative if something makes them angry. They can be equally committed to wreaking vengeance in a sharp and hurtful way. Everything has a purpose, including their friendships. Passion may run so high that they are intolerant of anyone who gets in their way, not hesitating to 'burn' them if it suits their purpose.

Kapha individuals are, on the whole, calm, peaceful
and reliable people who are most at ease in the cosy
environment of home and family. Unfortunately, some of
these characteristics may lead, in excess, to idleness,
addiction, jealousy and selfishness. However, these people
usually have personalities that are rock solid, so stable that
they may appear to be inactive in both mind and body.
They usually take an inordinate amount of time to start an
activity but will see it through to the end with stubborn
determination, regardless of difficulties. This aspect is true
of every branch of their lives; friendships form slowly, but
persist to the grave.

Please tick the feature below which *most* describes you.

Characteristic	*Vata*	*Pitta*	*Kapha*
Personality	❏ Uncertain, changeable, short relationships	❏ Passionate, brave, purposeful relationships	❏ Calm, reliable, stubborn, lasting relationships

ORGANISATION AND DAILY ROUTINE

Vata characters are the antithesis of creatures of habit.
They never keep good records and money-wise are always
in a mess. The normal routines of life such as eating,
drinking and sleeping happen with little apparent pattern
except that imposed by society and circumstance. Their
houses are generally disorganised, with the things they
might need tomorrow left out 'just in case'.

Pitta people are the planners and organisers of this
world. They are financially well organised, work out what
they can afford to spend and do it very sensibly. They are
not creatures of habit, but use their habits for their own

ends, modifying them as they go along. Their homes are neat and tidy in a purposeful way — they know where everything is and why.

Kapha people are almost exclusively creatures of habit. They revel in habits to the point that they often get stuck in a groove like a record on an old gramophone. They are financially prudent and always have resources put by for a rainy day. When taken to extremes they may appear to spend little and infrequently. Their homes are a picture of compulsive neatness. Nothing is thrown away, everything is stored in case it is needed one day.

Please tick the feature below which *most* describes you.

Characteristic	*Vata*	*Pitta*	*Kapha*
Organisation#	❑ Disorganised, difficulty sticking to routines	❑ Neat, tidy and purposeful	❑ Very neat, storing everything away for a rainy day
Finances#	❑ Impulse buying, financial chaos	❑ Clear financial planning, purposeful buying	❑ Saver, tends not to spend

SUMMARIES OF CONSTITUTIONAL TYPES

Add up the number of ticks you have for each of the categories *vata*, *pitta* and *kapha* in answering the questions above. Usually, one or two will have a clearly higher total than the others. These higher totals indicate what sort of basic constitution you have — your *prakruti*. For example, if you counted approximately twelve vatas/twenty-four pittas/four kaphas, your basic constitution is probably predominantly *pitta* with an element of *vata* (*pitta-vata*). If

you counted three vatas/thirty-four pittas/three kaphas,
your constitution is predominately *pitta*. If there is an even
balance between the three doshas, then add up again but
using only those ticks with a '#' beside them. This should
give you a clear view of the balance of the doshas in your
constitution.

Below are summaries of the various constitutional
types in general terms. No account has been taken of the
predominance of one characteristic over another when
two doshas predominate over the third. For example,
twelve vatas, twenty-four pittas, four kaphas and twenty-
four vatas, twelve pittas, four kaphas both represent *pitta-
vata* constitutions and are dealt with by a single summary
below.

However, in the former case there will be a tendency
towards *pitta* and thus the *pitta* summary should be read as
well; and in the latter case a tendency towards *vata*, in
which case understanding will be helped by reading the
vata summary in combination with *pitta-vata*. Listed first
are the simple types where one *dosha* is much more
evident than the other two and then those mixtures (most
of us) where one *dosha* is clearly much less evident than
the other two.

VATA

Vata people are usually rather thin and do not gain weight
easily, except when they over indulge in food. They have
narrow shoulders and hips and their joints tend to make
cracking noises when flexed. They find it hard to sit still.
They have dry rough skin which chaps easily and is also
prone to corns and calluses. Similarly, the hair tends to be
coarse, dry and curly. They suffer from the cold and
frequently complain of poor circulation in the extremities.

The skin is often cool to the touch, they have scanty sweat and enjoy a warm climate, preferably full sunlight.

The appetite is unpredictable; it is easily affected by over indulgence in activities that are exciting or absorbing to the point that eating is forgotten, sometimes resulting in further damage to the digestion. Dietary preferences are akin to the love of certain types of weather — vatas adore hot food.

Their ability to do things is variable, due to extreme fluctuations of their energy levels, related to their irregular eating and sleeping habits. The *vata* person keeps going, despite needing to take a rest, by consuming large quantities of tea and coffee. Not recognising this leads to continued frenetic activity, followed by exhaustion, and reinforces the pattern of life that typifies the *vata* individual. Despite the tendency to reach the stage of utter fatigue, they often have difficulty falling asleep, or once asleep they continually wake and fall asleep, often over sleeping in the morning. They can reach such a level of exhaustion that they sleep as if comatose.

Sensations tend to be excessively appreciated; they are typically nervous and jumpy. The sound of a door slamming will cause them to jump out of their skins and they may over-react to painful stimuli. The need to reduce this type of over-stimulation may express itself in the *vata* person as fear. Soothing music, soft oily massage and a quiet, warm environment without extremes are what these people prefer.

The lack of habitual routines in life leads to chaos in their lifestyle. If absence of control and peace typifies your life, then you almost certainly have *vata* as your key predominant *dosha*.

PITTA

Pitta people are well built and well proportioned. They
have regular, hearty appetites and their eating habits are
well planned. Weight can be gained if there is over-eating,
but this is unusual. They are intense people, sometimes to
the extent of being seen as sharp, irritable or intolerant.
Red, the colour of fire, characterises these individuals,
resulting in fair skin, often with freckles and moles. They
blush easily and also burn readily in the sun, which tends
to amplify the freckles. The hair is generally straight, fair
or red in colour, indeed, anyone who has red hair has *pitta*
as a significant element of their *prakruti*. They sweat
readily, because of all the heat stored inside.

*Pitta*s have razor sharp minds and are usually witty.
Because of this and the hot, intense nature of fire, they do
not tolerate fools gladly. They tend towards impatience.
They usually sleep soundly, because it is part of their
'plan'. They apply the same passion and ambition to all
they do, at work or play. They will see a task through to its
end with a purposeful approach. *Pitta* types prefer cool,
well structured environments.

KAPHA

The *kapha* person is normally large framed, with natural
athletic skills, especially while at school. The problem,
however, tends to be that they gain weight just by looking
at food, especially if not exercising. This leads to a loss of
athletic ability as the years go by. The majority of people
with a *kapha* constitution are healthy most of the time, but
over-eating may cause illness which is out of character
with their nature.

Kaphas have heavy emotional needs and frequently
fulfill these by using food as a substitute. Their innate

feeling of hunger, however, is never as intense as that of the *pitta* person, and always more regular than that of the *vata* individual. It is the need for emotional satisfaction that modifies the appetite and leads to a paradoxically high appetite. *Kapha* people are often a serious mix of paradoxes. They sleep very soundly and have a natural tendency to oversleep.

They are laid-back people who, on the whole, do not hunger after the same degree of excitement and arousal that *vata* and *pitta* people love. Once aroused, however, their appetites — for sex, for example — may become very strong. They are slow to rouse, but then the athletic nature breaks through and will maintain their drive to reach the end. *Kapha* people are stable, outwardly somewhat slow, and may appear to be complacent. They are creatures of habit and may become stuck in a rut because the environment they have is so enjoyable that they resist change and may become greedy, obdurate or overtly reactionary.

DUAL CONSTITUTIONS

If you have just one predominant *dosha*, you know how you are going to react to any situation. However, if you have more than one, you can never be absolutely sure which *dosha* is going to be most influential in any particular circumstance. In one situation, one *dosha* will be important in gauging your response, in another situation it will be the alternative. These constitutions are mixtures of *vata* and *pitta*, *kapha* and *pitta* or *vata* and *kapha* and you will probably fit into one of these categories. The examples below are very general, and cannot take account of the fact that as an individual you will probably have a somewhat different balance than the example quoted — so do not expect a complete match.

Vata-Pitta (or Pitta-Vata)

These people often have the cold hands and feet that
are the bane of the *vata* individual's life. They also love
warm climates, despite the *pitta* element in their make-up.
The *pitta* influence, however, does limit the degree of
heat they feel comfortable with. They love to eat but
have great difficulty in digesting food properly, especially
raw food.

In many areas of the outward signs of their
constitution they show combined characteristics. For
example, the combination of the curly hair of the *vata*
character and the straight hair of the *pitta* individual leads
frequently to wavy hair. More frequently, the effects of *vata*
and *pitta* appear predominately in different areas of the
individual. Furthermore, the two doshas can alternate with
each other depending upon the circumstances. Thus a
vata-pitta type can feel insecure in one confrontational
situation and yet on another day experience severe anger
at the same type of situation; it depends upon the balance
within the person at the time. Worst of all, both may be
present almost simultaneously, so that the person knows
what to do to solve a particular problem, but then feels
insecure about the ability to actually do it.

This duality can, nonetheless, be the *vata-pitta* person's
greatest asset if properly directed. Imagine the *vata* ability
for original thought and spontaneity, combined with the
passion and application of *pitta*. It is a combination that is
without equal, but it needs proper direction. Without
balance it can lead to frenetic attachment to sensual
pleasure as the source of fulfilment; it is the opportunity
for development of self awareness that must be explored,
for this will create the stability that this character type so
desperately needs.

Pitta-Kapha (or Kapha-Pitta)

The combination of the stability of *kapha* together with *pitta*'s ability to accommodate change results in a personality that is perhaps more capable than most in coping with our turbulent world. There is, of course, a down-side which is a combination of the self-satisfied smugness of the *kapha* individual together with the superior and egotistical nature of the *pitta* person. These people can become wrapped up in their own little world to the total exclusion of others — they can be impossible to live with!

However, they are often successful people. The power and enthusiasm of the *pitta* is expressed superbly in *kapha*'s solid physique; the balance of emotions is such that they are slow to anger, unlike pure *pitta*s, but do not store emotions for too long, unlike the pure *kapha*. Climate is of little concern to them, as they have the ability to cope with both extremes of hot and cold.

Owing to their low inherent *vata*, *pitta-kapha* types need to achieve balance by spiritual exploration and discipline. They also need to be 'kicked' by unusual situations occasionally in order to prevent the smug over-confidence that can be their hallmark.

Vata-Kapha (or Kapha-Vata)

This combination can be the most difficult to deal with because of the extreme opposite nature of the two doshas involved. The doshas do have one thing in common, a propensity for coldness — they lack fire. The insulating qualities of *kapha* tend to prevent this as a perceived symptom. The difficulties that arise do so because of the lack of fire more than anything else. This low fire (or *agni*) means they tend to have digestive problems. They are not

able to digest food fully and so the bowel itself will be
poorly nourished, leading to gassy indigestion and
frequent bouts of constipation mixed with occasional
diarrhoea. The other important area affected by the lack of
fire is in the emotional world. They have a very high level
of need for emotional fire to be supplied by someone else.

Kapha-vata types are generally tall, but of average
build. They do most things in earnest but sometimes make
the *vata* mistake of not applying measure to their efforts.
This can be most damaging when their desires on an
emotional level are frustrated; they impose a level of hurt
upon themselves which is located very deeply and tends
never to be forgotten. It is a feature of the indiscretion of
the *vata* and elephantine memory of the *kapha*.

They are excellent examples of the potential for
alternation of characteristics in people ruled by two
doshas. They can be fancy-free one minute, yet profound
and secretive the next.

THE MEANING OF YOUR *PRAKRUTI*

You should not view the above analysis as an attempt to fit
you and your constitution into a box — nothing could be
further from the truth. The concept of constitutional types
is basically straightforward, though it may not seem so
right now. It will become clearer as you observe the way
you live in this world. We all have a body and mind quite
unlike that of any other person, although ultimately the
central light within us all that is our 'self' *is* identical. It is
simply the body and mind which differ from person to
person and which need to be kept in balance to achieve
perfect health. The exercise of finding out which
constitutional type you are does not bind you to one
stereotype; it provides you with information on qualities

which are so deeply intrinsic in you that they must be consciously balanced. It provides a simple foundation on which you can work to create a new, balanced healthy you.

Remember that your assessment of your constitution is affected to some extent by that very constitution. This is not a problem — it simply means that some of your perceptions of yourself may not be absolutely accurate at the moment. As you come into a better state of balance with yourself, it will be more apparent what the accurate answers are and thus it is important to revisit this chapter perhaps every three months to reassess your *prakruti*. Try to do this as if for the first time, each time; it will not be easy, but will reap worthwhile rewards in the long run.

CHAPTER SIX

Treatment with Ayurveda

According to ayurvedic teaching, starting any form of treatment without first dealing with the toxins in the system that have caused the disease will only make matters worse. In the short term, treatment may superficially relieve the symptoms, but the imbalance in the doshas will manifest as disease again either in the same location or elsewhere. Toxins may either be eliminated or neutralised. This applies to both the physical and emotional level of disease.

THE EMOTIONAL LEVEL

Anxiety, anger, fear, insecurity, jealousy and greed are human emotions recognised by us all, but we are taught as children that it is not appropriate to express these 'negative' feelings. Ayurveda teaches us that this is incorrect thinking and that it is important to release these emotions; otherwise imbalance in the doshas will occur, leading to a build up of disease-creating toxins.

First of all, we need to know what our repressed emotions are. Sometimes they have been so effectively buried that we are quite unaware of them. The only way to find out is by observation. This is a little more than plain observation of what is going on in our lives — it involves observing the observer, even though that sounds almost impossible. It helps to ask the question: 'Who is it that observes you are happy (or sad or angry, etc.)'?; 'Who is it that is aware you are seeing this page'? The answer is the true self, or the soul, unchangeable and unaffected by the exigencies of life; in western medicine it is sometimes referred to as insight — literally looking inwards.

There are many techniques you can use to assist in this process of observation. It helps to pause for a couple of seconds before doing anything; discussion with a group of like-minded individuals refines the ability to make contact with this insight; meditation is extremely useful. See Helpful Addresses for information on organisations that will assist you if you wish to follow this path.

Observation is the key to understanding your emotions. For example, if anger arises, you should be completely aware of it — do not try to do anything about it, just observe. In this way, you will learn how it arose and what it resulted in. Release of anger is the important feature and, once again, this involves not doing anything; simple observation will enable its release.

The Physical Level
Diet

The guiding principle of Ayurveda is that each person has the power to heal herself. Much can be done to remove or neutralise toxins in the body by balancing the doshas, using an appropriate diet as part of a programme of measure in all aspects of life. Such dietary adjustments will also serve to maintain the balance of the doshas and thus perfect health. Spiritual development is vitally important, but it is difficult to maintain if the body and mind are ailing, so our eating habits must be examined.

What is eaten should be chosen to balance the individual constitution. Choosing the proper diet is a simple matter, given an understanding of the constitution and how it relates to the qualities of various foods. The taste of the food (sweet, sour, salty, pungent, bitter or

astringent) and the season of the year must also be
considered.

You should not eat unless you are feeling hungry, nor
drink unless you are feeling thirsty. Do not confuse these
two feelings; it is a great temptation to drink in order to
assuage hunger, but all that will happen is the digestive fire
will be diluted.

In the process of eating, you are feeding not just the
body but the mind and spirit as well. It is important
therefore, to feed all five of the senses by preparing and
consuming food which is attractive to look at, good to
taste, inspiring to smell, pleasant in constitution. It may
seem difficult to satisfy the sense of hearing, but the sound
of food being cooked or of a stick of raw celery being
chewed can do so in a very pleasing way.

Always prepare food, serve it and eat it with love.
We have all had the experience that food cooked by
someone who loves us is somehow more pleasing than
that cooked without love. To hold on to unloving feelings
while we are eating tends to cause indigestion. Poor
digestion will give rise to production of *ama* and thus
to the promotion of disease. Drink water with your
meal in sips. After you have finished eating, a mixture
of yogurt and water will aid digestion. This drink should
be about half yogurt and half water, but see what suits
you best. If you have *vata* as a strong characteristic, then
add a little lemon juice. If your major *dosha* is *pitta*, then
add a little sugar. For *kapha* individuals, a little honey
and a sprinkle of fresh black pepper is probably a good
idea. This is specifically a drink for the end of, rather
than during, a meal. The best drink during the meal
itself is water; don't drink milk with a meal, especially
if the food contains meat.

Allow your food to pass well down the digestive system before taking any strenuous exercise if possible. When you exercise, the body reduces the blood supply to the gut and makes it available to the appropriate muscles; this disrupts the whole process of digestion and must be avoided if *ama* is not to be produced. The same is true of sleeping; the circulation of blood in the body changes profoundly and the gut is no longer supplied with what it needs to allow correct digestion and assimilation of what you have just eaten. Avoid both these 'activities' for a good two hours after a meal. This does not mean that you cannot, though, go for a stroll after eating — it is almost certainly beneficial to take a gentle walk following a meal.

Food has the property, as far as digestion is concerned, of being either heavy or light, related largely to the amount of digestion required. So light foods include cooked rice and potatoes, whereas heavy foods include things like raw food and cooked meat. We tend to think, in the west, that salads are 'light' food, but actually they require a lot more digestion than a cooked vegetable. Raw and cooked food have different amounts of *agni* present in them and should never be eaten in the same meal, except in very small quantities.

Light food makes it easier to integrate body, mind and spirit, because there is less re-distribution of blood to the gut for digestion. Heavy food always leaves you feeling tired and lethargic, often actually inducing sleep.

Diet and the Mind
Everything you eat will affect your mind as well as your body. In Ayurveda, the mind has three possible states, which are related to the state of the constitution as a whole:

- *sattva*, or peaceful equilibrium, in which the power
  of discrimination is most accessible
- *rajas*, or activity, in which excessive thoughts
  prevent discrimination from being accessed
- *tamas*, or inertia, in which there is a heaviness and
  attachment to the physical realm such that there is
  neither activity nor discrimination.

This division of states of mind is the cause of another of
those vicious circles that tend to characterise our lives.
The power of discrimination allows us to know the
correct balance and what is the most appropriate action in
a certain situation. If this is clouded or access to it is not
possible, then we are unable to decide, for example, what
to eat and how much; this can give rise to a more tamasic
state, which further obscures discrimination!

Food which is bad, fermented or preserved for too
long increases the amount of *tamas* in the body and so in
the mind. A good example of a fermented food is alcohol.
This does not mean we should not drink alcohol, but we
are all aware of the effects of too much! Legumes and
high-protein food like meat, fish, and poultry increase
rajas, as do any of the pungent spices. To increase *sattva,*
we should increase our intake of grains, fruits and most
vegetables.

Dos and Don'ts

Always eat fresh foods when possible and avoid preserved,
canned or even frozen food items, though the latter are
permissible if fresh is not available. Eat light foods until
your appetite is satisfied, but do not be tempted to clear
the plate just because there is food on it. With heavy
foods, try to restrict yourself to satisfying only half your
appetite with this type of ingredient. If you are ill, eat only

light foods, and then in small quantities, until half your
appetite — at the most — is fulfilled.

One of the most important rules in Ayurveda is never
to combine in one meal foods which 'fight', either in
terms of the signals they give to the gut or in terms of
their qualities:

- do not eat cooked foods and raw foods at the same
  meal as they require different types of digestion
- avoid combining heavy and light foods
- avoid drinking milk while eating radishes, tomatoes,
  potatoes, bananas, meat, fish, eggs, citrus fruits,
  melon, bread or cherries
- do not mix milk and yoghurt
- always eat fresh fruit separately from your meals
  (cooked fruit may be eaten at the same time as a
  cooked meal)
- avoid mixing different types of protein, such as meat
  and cheese.

In recent years, western medical research has identified
other unhelpful food combinations in line with the
traditional ayurvedic ones above. Keep heavy high protein
or high fat food items in separate meals from lighter foods
such as starches and vegetables. These types of food
require quite different digestive processes in the gut for
proper nutrition. If you eat them together, there will be
competition for the appropriate digestive mechanism and
neither will be digested properly. Proteins and fats require
slow digestion and absorption by the small bowel, whereas
starches need to pass quickly to the large bowel, where
they are acted upon by bacteria to produce special forms
of food. Your small bowel needs this form of food. If they
are eaten together, then fat and protein slow down the
passage of the starches and they do not reach the large

bowel in time to be digested by this special bacterial
mechanism. It is your bowel or gut that suffers and is
unable to function properly as the controller of food
entering the body.

Do your best to maintain the separations between
different types of foods as indicated above — there is
nothing 'wrong' with any of them, they just do not
combine well.

Taste

All foods have their own 'taste' characteristics, which
interact with your body and your consciousness. These
effects are complex and not necessarily obvious. Take a
little piece of raw potato and chew it in the mouth for
four or five minutes. Observe the way that the taste
changes as it is chewed; it begins by tasting rather dry and
almost astringent, but after a while it starts to taste sweet.
This is because it is being partly digested in your mouth,
which makes it sweet tasting.

Understanding a particular food, taste, energy and
post-digestive effect makes it easier to see how it is going
to interact with your mind and body, but it can be difficult
to remember all these influences. In appendices *Vata*, *Pitta*
and *Kapha*, pages 101–15, you will find listed foods which
may be eaten by people of various constitutions together
with a list of those that should not be, because of their
tendency to aggravate the predominant *dosha* and create
imbalance.

DUAL CONSTITUTIONS

If like most people you have two predominant doshas in
your basic constitution, then read the following sections
bearing in mind the comments below. You will also by

now have some idea which of the doshas in your mind and body are out of balance; you should apply the dietary rules appropriate for the *dosha* which is out of balance.

The following sections make reference to environmental factors, the chief among these being the effects of the seasons upon your present balance. Spring and summer are warm times, characterised by growth and activity. As a result, there is a natural increase of *pitta* in the constitutional balance and if this is your predominant *dosha* you will need to pay extra attention to keeping it under control. This applies equally to the other doshas; autumn is a time of increased *vata*, when winds are high, leaves are falling off the trees and everything is drying out. The depth of winter and the early part of spring are times when *kapha* is increased. We already tend to modify our diets naturally, by eating salads in the summer, and hot soup on a cold winter night *feels* just right!

VATA-PITTA

The external influences which affect your balance are the presence of increased *vata* in the environment in autumn and winter and excess *pitta* in the spring and summer. So, as a general rule you should follow the dietary advice for *vata* during autumn and winter, followed by the advice for *pitta* during the spring and summer. In each case, the dietary recommendations given in the appendices will help to keep each list's *dosha* under control.

Pungent tastes increase both *vata* and *pitta* doshas in the individual and the taste of sweet foods reduces both, so you should avoid spicy, pungent food, however much you may be tempted. Try to keep your diet high in sweet items (sweet here means the ultimate effect of the taste, not necessarily the taste when you first put the food in your mouth).

PITTA-KAPHA

Because there are external environmental factors, similar
to those for the *vata-pitta* person, affecting your mind and
body, you should use the dietary advice given for *pitta*
during the spring and summer, followed by the *kapha*
dietary recommendations during autumn and winter. The
food tastes you should avoid, because they aggravate both
pitta and *kapha*, are sour and salty. The tastes that are good
for you are essentially bitter and astringent.

VATA-KAPHA

As a result of external environmental factors affecting your
mind and body, use the dietary advice for *vata* during the
summer and autumn, together with that for *kapha* during
the winter and spring months. Make sure that during the
summer you have some sweet foods to help balance the
vata and that during the winter there are elements of bitter
and astringent tastes to balance the *kapha*.

VATA INDIVIDUALS

Try to eat little and often; three or preferably four times a
day. You may also eat snacks in between meals, but be sure
to allow the previous meal to pass well into the digestive
system before consuming the next one. Allow at least two
hours between meals or snacks. If you eat more frequently,
your gut will still be in the appropriate state for digesting
the previous food and will not be ready to start dealing
with the next input.

You will do best with cooked food; keep raw food to
a minimum and at all costs avoid fried foods. The variable
nature of the digestion in *vata* people means that there is a
particular problem with the digestive process if foods of
markedly differing heaviness, or raw and cooked, are

combined. The gut needs a clear signal as to which type of food it is going to be dealing with, or it becomes confused and agitated. This is why separating raw and cooked food is much more important for pure *vata* types than others.

The *vata* person's diet should also be as regular as possible, as irregularity will aggravate *vata* and add to the problem of poor digestion. It should be as balanced as possible, with no excess of any particular food type, as *vata* is always aggravated by excess. Try to avoid foods which have bitter, pungent or astringent tastes.

Any sweetener may be used sparingly in cooking/food preparation, although white sugar should never be used. Avoid bread which has been made with yeast because the gassy nature of the yeast will increase *vata*; however, as all bread is somewhat dry and has some sort of gas-producing mechanism in its production, it should only be eaten in moderation.

All vegetables must be cooked and those in the list (Appendix *Vata*) to be avoided are permissible to eat, if cooked and not consumed too frequently. If you feel like a salad occasionally, then make sure it is covered with plenty of sweet, oily dressing. Fruits permitted for the *vata* individual must never be eaten in a dried form, for example, dried apricots. Eat them stewed or fresh occasionally. Avoid fruit that is unripe — it tends to be astringent, especially bananas.

You can benefit from a small amount of meat in your diet, but see the list for which are recommended and which are prohibited. If you eat meat excessively, it will weaken your digestion, though in small quantities it is useful because of the complete protein balance that it provides, plus its 'grounding' effect.

All beans should be eaten in moderation, for they are high in protein and will lead to an increase of gaseous nitrogenous waste products if consumed in excess. The *vata* nature of these proteins can be reduced to some extent by soaking them before cooking and discarding the water; then cooking in fresh water. The presence of ginger or garlic when cooking them can increase *agni* and reduce the gas producing tendency, as can adding a little oil. It is best to experiment and see what technique produces least gas in the gut.

Provided you do not have a dairy allergy, dairy products are good for you — with the proviso that hard cheeses should be eaten sparingly.

Vata people often like hot spices, but beware their tendency to aggravate *vata* in the long run. Also, if you have a significant element of *pitta* in your constitution, then the spices will be disastrous in their effect on the *pitta dosha*. Your naturally addictive personality will strongly crave nicotine, white sugar and caffeine if exposed to them; avoid them at all costs. Alcohol in moderation is of benefit to the *vata* person; but 'moderation' is the key word.

PITTA INDIVIDUALS

You should eat three well defined meals per day, with a gap of at least four and preferably six hours between them. You may have snacks, but leave a gap of three hours between your meals and your snacks. Avoid fried foods, because the process of frying adds intense heat to the food and this can de-stabilise *pitta*. Raw foods are good for you and your digestion has enough *agni* to be able to deal with them. Cooked foods will tend to increase *pitta* too much if you are not careful.

Avoid hot tastes — sour, salty or pungent — in your
food and place emphasis in your diet on the sweet, bitter
and astringent tastes. Specific foods to avoid are: meat,
eggs, salt and alcohol. Vegetables, grain, and fruit, as listed
in Appendix *Pitta*, are the best foods for you. Largely
yours should be a vegetarian diet; however, there are a few
meats listed in the appendix which can be eaten
infrequently and in small quantity without too much
harm.

Avoid bread which has been made with yeast because
of the sour nature of the fermentation process. Non-yeast
or unleavened breads are excellent for you. Vegetables can
be eaten raw, and should be consumed frequently, but
avoid hot vegetables such as radish and peppers. Generally,
red vegetables — for example, tomatoes — are forbidden.

Remember to select fruit that is sweet and avoid those
that are sour — this may apply simply to how ripe
something is, so do not eat a fruit on the recommended
list if it is unripe. Citrus fruits in small quantities reduce
pitta because their post-digestive effect is not heating unless
consumed in large quantities. This is because the acid in
them is capable of being removed easily from the body, via
the lungs as carbon dioxide, thus leaving *anti-pitta* residue.

Meat should be avoided, especially seafood, which is
said to be 'hot' and can cause allergies. Egg yolks are hot
and egg whites cooling, so eggs need to be separated into
their component parts and the yolk thrown away most of
the time! You have the luxury of being able to digest
almost anything, but beware of beans in too large a
quantity; the same waste products that affect *vata*
individuals so badly also aggravate the *pitta dosha*.

If you eat a vegetarian diet, be careful to avoid nuts
and oils in general. These are too heating for the *pitta*

person with one or two exceptions, especially coconut,
which has a very cooling effect. All dairy products —
milk, unsalted butter, cream and soft cheese — are
excellent. To avoid the negative tastes above, you should
steer clear of hard cheeses, salted butter and yoghurt,
unless it has had some fire, such as cinnamon, added to it
and has been diluted at least half and half with water. Any
sweetener can be used (including white sugar) but not
molasses or honey, both of which are hot. Hot spices are
guaranteed to increase the *pitta* part of your nature and a
careful choice of cooling herbs should be made. The *pitta*
individual should never add salt to her food.

KAPHA INDIVIDUALS

A *kapha* person should eat only two meals a day, allowing
at least a six-hour gap between them. You should not take
snacks in between. You will have a natural tendency to be
able to eat as much as you feel like and so consciously
need to make an effort to limit the total amount you eat at
each meal. There is a relatively low amount of digestive
fire, or *agni*, and you should generally stick to cooked
food. Occasional consumption of raw foods will help to
clean the gut, but over indulgence will cause digestive
problems because of the lack of intrinsic fire. As for the
other doshas, fried foods should always be avoided,
because the heaviness of the fat will tend to aggravate the
kapha dosha.

   You need to pay attention in your diet to bitter,
pungent and astringent foods. You need to avoid the
sweet, sour and salty food elements and you should stay
clear of dairy products altogether. If you wish to eat grains
of any sort, or bread, make sure the grains are roasted or
the bread toasted. You need 'heat' in your foods and the

grains listed in Appendix *Kapha* have been selected with this in mind. Different types of grain have different amounts of intrinsic heat within them; wheat, for instance, is very heavy, oily and cold, and should therefore be avoided.

All vegetables are good for you, with the exception of potatoes, tomatoes and water chestnuts. You can eat as many vegetables as often as you like, but remember not to have them raw except occasionally. Root vegetables tend to be sweet, and thus should take second place to those growing above ground. The fruits you eat should be 'dry', like apples, and not those that are full of water or which are very sweet or very sour.

Try to stay away from meat, but if you feel the need to eat it, make sure it is dry roasted or grilled; never have fried meat — you do not need its grounding effect. Stick to the list recommended in Appendix *Kapha*. The same principles apply to the various beans that are available; you do not need very much of them, so restrict your intake and stay away from the heavier varieties such as kidney beans. If you do have beans, eat them in small quantities.

Nuts and seeds contain large amounts of oils and are definitely not for you. In fact you should avoid oils of all sorts, as previously mentioned. This applies also to dairy products, which you should steer well clear of. Do not use sweet substances of any sort, under any circumstances.

Hot spices are an excellent idea in an attempt to increase the innate fire of the food you are eating. It is difficult for you to use too much!

CHAPTER SEVEN

Your Weight and Ayurveda

The consumer-driven world in which we live constantly urges us to consume. The Health of The Nation targets exhort us to lose weight by reducing the amount of fat and salt in our diets. Yet the food industry adds salt, sugar and fat to all processed foods, often to mask the poor taste of the ingredients or to create taste where none exists. There are other ways of adding flavour to prepared food, but these are expensive. So it is hardly surprising that despite all the good intentions of weight reduction programmes, aimed at improving our health, we are still becoming more and more overweight.

If you are of a predominantly *vata* constitution and you are overweight, then it is simply because you eat too much, or you may need to review your constitution to see if you have more *kapha* in your *prakruti* than you thought. *Pitta* people can gain weight easily, especially from overeating, but they also tend to be able to lose it readily. If you have a *kapha* constitution, there are two important things to be aware of: firstly, you will always have a well rounded body (this does not mean obese) and you will never be able to — nor should you try to — achieve a thin, 'super-model' image. Secondly, you will put on weight easily and will tend to hang on to it. This is true also for the *pitta-kapha* constitution. If you are *vata-pitta*, you will tend to have the same characteristic ability to gain and lose weight as the *pitta* individual. If you have *vata-kapha* characteristics, whilst you will find it difficult to lose weight, it also goes on quite slowly.

WHY ARE WE OVERWEIGHT?

We eat because we are told to; this was the case when we were children and now as adults by advertising. We also eat as a substitute for love, or as a way of trying to rectify imbalances in our doshas, especially on the emotional level — fear, insecurity, anger or depression. These are partially solvable by diet, but it is more important to solve the problem that is causing the emotion in the first place. This latter aspect of treatment is in our own hands, but is not easy to approach and so it is important to seek professional help from an ayurvedic practitioner. Failing this, seek the support of your partner or best friend and listen to what they say. Try not to use food as a substitute.

Also, because processed foods are packed with salt, sugar and fat, make your own meals from fresh ingredients and do not use these additives. Do not buy processed foods or snacks, or even a ready-made sandwich unless it is labelled 'no added salt' and 'low fat' If you tend to buy snacks for lunch, try buying a freshly made sandwich (while you wait) so you can determine what goes into it — it is just about to go into *you*! Buy a banana, apple, orange or other fresh fruit, depending upon which are recommended in the list for your *dosha*.

DIETS

Simple calorie-controlled diets are inappropriate for modifying weight and yet many people are addicted to them. Reduced calorie intake is beneficial, but what is important is the *way* we reduce the calories and the reasons for doing so. Too often, the desire to 'go on a diet' represents a form of self-punishment because we feel guilty about our current body image. This is not a helpful attitude.

Crash diets usually represent a desire to lose weight rapidly. Remember that our weight and the ratio of fat in our bodies has built up over many years, and expecting it to disappear in a few days or weeks is *not* realistic. If we starve ourselves (often the essential goal of a strict calorie controlled diet) the weight will surely vanish; but by doing this, we lose something called 'lean body mass', the muscles and other tissues that make up the body and consume most of the calories we eat most of the time. If we lose lean body mass, then when the diet stops as inevitably it will, we tend to return to what we were eating before and the weight goes back on faster than ever. This is because our energy expenditure, or basal metabolic rate (BMR), is now less than it was before the diet started, because of the reduction in lean body mass.

Don't expect to lose more than 1 lb/½ kg every week on average. In fact, you should only measure your weight once a week, at the same time of the same day of the week each time, and even then only gauge whether you are actually losing weight once a month. This is because body weight varies naturally from one end of the day to the other and from day to day for all sorts of reasons, especially if you are a woman. One lb a week doesn't sound like very much — but think about it; that's 52 lbs/24 kg in a year.

Exercise is usually recommended by anyone advising a weight loss programme, but why? The reasons are three-fold. Moderate exercise, such as a brisk walk for thirty minutes five times per week, preferably daily, will burn off a few calories, but that is a relatively small effect — you won't notice any change in weight between the start and end of the walk!

Going for a brisk walk regularly has a much more important effect concerning the control of *vata,* which intrudes into the lives of all but a few of us. Analysis of our appetites shows that they vary from day to day between 2,000 and 5,000 calories, despite the fact that our energy expenditure is usually only about 2,500 calories! This is a typical *vata* characteristic, caused by our life styles. As energy expenditure by the individual increases towards 3,500 calories, the top end of the appetite range comes down to 3,500 calories, and from there on it goes up if energy expenditure goes up. Thus the effect of exercise on the appetite can be quite dramatic. Even deep remedial massage can have a similar effect.

Exercise helps to maintain, or even increase, lean body mass, so that your basal metabolic rate goes up — meaning it is more difficult to put weight on again. That said, of course, you are not going to stop the diet you are on because in Ayurveda you will simply have changed the *way* you eat.

There is also evidence that exercising and losing weight alters something called insulin sensitivity. Insulin is the most important hormone in the body concerned with the control of calories. As we become overweight, it seems that the sensitivity of our cells to insulin reduces, leading to additional problems with calorie intake and weight. By reducing overweight, the sensitivity to insulin returns towards normal. In extreme circumstances it is this loss of insulin sensitivity which gives rise to late onset diabetes. So there are many good reasons for exercising, not just to burn calories.

AYURVEDIC CONTROL OF BODY WEIGHT

The principle of ayurvedic therapy is to pay attention to balancing the doshas, which constitute who and how you are today, on the surface, and to give the correct signals to the gut. The gut, or more properly the entire digestive tract, is the central control system for our bodies in terms of the food we eat; it even contains the cells that manufacture insulin, embedded in the pancreas. So if we give it signals that are at odds with reality, it becomes confused and is unable to apply the correct measures to ensure efficient digestion and absorption.

In addition to the exercises mentioned above, you need to stop eating the foods which are on the 'No' list in Appendix *Kapha*. This is true whatever your basic constitution, except that if you are a pure *vata* person then you will need to balance this with the foods which you are recommended to eat in the *vata* list to maintain control of your *vata*. The important rule to remember is never to combine foods which fight, because they require different types of digestion for a healthy gut.

Also, bear in mind that whilst high protein diets are used by some people for weight reduction, they are not particularly pleasant, largely because the sweet taste is completely absent from the food. So always have some complex carbohydrate (soluble fibre) in your diet; your large bowel needs it to stay healthy, and keep it separate from the protein. Avoid salty tastes.

Signals to the gut are extremely important. You should avoid ice cold food and drinks at all cost. If the stomach senses 'cold' to that degree, it will assume that the external weather is cold and react by giving instructions to lay down fat as an insulator against the perceived weather, thus increasing the appetite. We all create this confusion in our intestines every time we eat ice-cream in the middle of summer or through having ice in our drinks. If you are on a weight-loss programme, then all drinks should be warm if possible and it does no harm to add an extra bit of 'heat' by drinking ginger tea. Just make an infusion of fresh or powdered ginger in some boiling water and drink that regularly. Eat all your food slowly; this will ensure that your mind receives the full taste of the food via the senses. Taste is as important a part of nourishment as the food itself in the ayurvedic system.

If you are a *kapha* or *pitta-kapha*, you tend to put on weight by looking at food. There is a good reason for this. When you look at something and crave it, the signal the gut and body receive from the mind tells them to get ready for calorific intake, and existing sugars in the blood stream are converted to storage elements such as glycogen and fat. Then all that happens is you feel hungry! So, try to stop looking at or fantasising about foods you are not going to eat.

How to Eat

In our western society, learning how to eat requires a change in thinking. We are taught to feel guilty about being overweight, but you should try to discard this emotion if you can. Decide from the advice above and the information given under Balancing the Doshas (page 116) which sort of dietary adjustment you are going to make; then stick to it, except for one meal a week when you may indulge yourself with whatever you wish. Be assured, this will make almost no difference to the course you have chosen, as long as you follow one vitally important rule — do not feel guilty about it. If you do, then you will come to regard the dietary balance you have chosen as a punishment. It is anything but a punishment and should be enjoyable.

Lastly, be aware of what you are eating at all times and when the feeling of hunger has gone, stop eating. Do not be tempted to clear your plate. We guarantee you will be surprised.

Chapter Eight

Obtaining Ayurvedic Care

I t is advisable to obtain advice from an ayurvedic physician to determine the exact nature of your constitution and the degree to which it is out of balance at present, especially if you are suffering overt symptoms of disease. The physician may give you advice on how to change your life style or your diet in order to alleviate your suffering. The added benefit is that the practitioner may detect imbalances you were unaware of, giving you the opportunity to re-balance these aspects *before* they cause a problem.

Your First Visit to a Practitioner

As in any valid medical system, the first thing that will happen, after you have been made comfortable, is that a history will be taken. In western medicine this usually concentrates more on your present circumstances than your past; in Ayurveda it tends to be the other way round. Also, you should expect questions about where you live now, or have lived in the past.

The practitioner will ask you many questions of the sort you have already answered in Chapter Five, in order to ascertain your *prakruti*. So even if you decide to follow the ayurvedic medical model just by visiting a practitioner and not by 'doing-it-yourself', you should still go through Chapter Five in detail, as many of the questions will be unfamiliar, especially if encountered for the first time in a consulting room. You may also be asked questions about your diet, so it is helpful to take along a list of *exactly* what you have eaten and drunk for the previous week. Do this as an exercise as the week goes by; do not try to do it at the end of a week from memory — for lots of reasons, it doesn't work.

THE EXAMINATION

Your practitioner will probably make a very detailed examination of your tongue. It carries a lot of information about the internal organs of your body and their state of health. It is traditional for a western medical doctor to ask to see your tongue, but only briefly; the ayurvedic practitioner will study it for longer.

You may be asked for a sample of your urine. If so, it will probably need to be an 'early morning' sample, so you will have to take it with you on your next visit.

Almost certainly, your practitioner will wish to take your pulse. In western medicine this appears to be a fairly straightforward process, but in fact it is quite complex, involving the speed, rhythm, force and shape of what is being felt; it tells the doctor a lot about your heart, blood vessels and general state of health. Your ayurvedic practitioner will wish to take your pulse at both of your wrists, probably simultaneously, using three fingers to do it each time; these are placed at the wrist in a special way, as explained earlier. Do not be surprised if your practitioner presses quite firmly with the fingers, because it is possible to assess not only your current doshic balance, but also your constitution and the status of the various organs in the body.

You will probably not even notice some of the examinations, especially that required for facial diagnosis, an important part of ayurvedic technique. But you will notice the examination of your nails, at least as important to the ayurvedic practitioner as to your 'western' doctor.

And you will not miss the fact that your eyes, or more
exactly your irises (the coloured part), are being
examined, as well as your conjunctivae (the white part).

THE COURSE OF TREATMENT

Your practitioner will explain to you your *prakruti* and
what the current state of balance implies, how imbalances
are causing the symptoms of disease that have brought you
to the consultation, and what to do to set the balance
right. Once the course of treatment/lifestyle/diet
modification has begun, your practitioner will want to
see you again, possibly quite regularly to begin with, to
make sure that the doshas are coming back into balance.
What is perhaps more important is that the practitioner
will be able to advise you in detail about the changes to
make in your life in the longer term to ensure good
health in the future.

SOME COMMON REMEDIES

DIZZINESS

Crush an onion and forcibly breathe in the aroma.

HEADACHE

Make a teaspoonful of ginger paste from dried powdered
ginger and water. Spread this on the inside of a length
of bandage sufficient to cover the forehead. Apply and
leave in position for an hour or so. Place 3 drops of
warm ghee in each nostril and sniff well to relieve tension.
Apply sesame oil (un-toasted) and massage into the
feet and the scalp. Apply pressure massage to both big
toes.

INSOMNIA

Apply sesame oil (un-toasted) to feet and scalp and
massage gently the centre of the forehead before retiring.
Drink almond milk, made as follows:
soak 10 almonds in warm water for 1–2 hours, then peel
place in a liquidiser/blender and add:
1 cup cow's milk
2 pinches nutmeg
1 pinch dried ginger
1 tsp ground cardamom
liquidise and drink before retiring.

RECEDING GUMS

At night, take a mouthful of warm, un-toasted sesame oil,
but do not swallow. After 5 minutes, spit it out and
massage the gums using the index finger. Use dental floss
to clean between the teeth. In the morning, chew a small
handful of sesame seeds.

Sometimes your physician may recommend certain special
ayurvedic treatments, some of which are described briefly
below.

MEDICINAL HERBS

There are many medicinal herbs and substances in the
ayurvedic pharmacy which may be used by your
practitioner to achieve various effects. Some are very
effective at creating balance within unbalanced doshas;
some are designed to eliminate *ama* that has accumulated
in a tissue. Make sure you know which manufacturer has
supplied your herbs and that they have been tested for the
presence of heavy metals.

SHIRODHARA

To the western mind, this treatment may seem somewhat
bizarre; it involves the continuous flow of warm oil over
the forehead. Strange though it may sound, it is extremely
relaxing and may dissolve deep seated emotional stress. It is
sometimes used as part of a more comprehensive treatment
known as *panchakarma*.

PANCHAKARMA

This is not a treatment for the faint-hearted. It involves
several days of preparation of the body with various forms
of deep massage, using a variety of oils, followed by a
purgative cleansing of the gut. It is extremely effective in
balancing the doshas and eliminating stored *ama*, but can
only be carried out by a qualified, experienced ayurvedic
physician.

FASTING

This process allows the body to digest and remove its *ama*
by itself. It must be undertaken only under the strict
supervision of an ayurvedic physician. The exact regimen
depends upon your constitution and may very probably
involve eating, but only one food, such as rice. It does not
necessarily mean eating or drinking nothing!

SWEATING

The physician may recommend, especially following oil
treatments, a period of forced sweating to help eliminate
ama and excess doshas. The methods are many and varied,
but all aim to achieve the same objective.

CHAPTER NINE

Case Studies

CASE ONE
MRS R.

Mrs R., a mother of four, was born in February 1920 and
has been a widow for twenty years. Her weight ranges
from 8 st 3 1bs to 8 st 12 1bs. She was born and lives in
Reading, Berkshire, which is damp, increasing her *kapha
dosha*. Her family history reveals a father who died of
pneumonia at the age of eighty-three. Her mother also
died of pneumonia, but had Alzheimer's disease as well.
All her cousins had asthma.

MEDICAL HISTORY

Her height of 5ft 2 in/1.57 m has decreased by 2in/5 cm
in six years due to osteoporosis, which is manifesting in
the spine as excessive curvature in both directions. Surgical
treatment has included removal of the gall-bladder in 1979
and an appendectomy, which results in a diminution of a
particular type of *pitta*. There is a history of diverticulitis,
hiatus hernia, kidney stones and sciatica on the right side
of the body, which disturbs her sleep. Heberden's nodules
are present in the joints of both hands and the feet display
osteoarthritic changes.

Mrs R.'s presenting symptoms are as follows: chronic
asthma from eight years of age, which kept her away from
school twenty-five per cent of the time. Allergens
identified which exacerbate the situation are animal hair,
house dustmite and feathers. The attacks ceased since oral
steroid therapy began twenty years ago.

THE EXAMINATION

Physical examination revealed a long-standing *vata* imbalance, the skin being fine, dry, cool and papery, prone to bruising and darkness, especially around the eyes. Her nails are ridged longitudinally with a loss of the moons, indicating a lung impairment. There is little or no hair on the body and the hair on the scalp has become progressively finer and finer. The eyes appear *pitta*, displaying a clear, steady gaze and the pupils also appear clear.

The tongue is deeply furrowed, narrow with two patches of froth over the lung areas. It also trembles uncontrollably, possibly indicating deep anxiety. Her bowel movements are regular. Her speech is sharp and staccato in nature. There would appear to be a decrease in the *udana* (or upward moving) *vata*, as her memory is very short. Mrs R. is on a cocktail of drugs, including prednisolone, which is being reduced *very* slowly.

It was important first to ascertain which type of asthma she was experiencing and it seems that it was a *vata* imbalance. The diverticulitis, hiatus hernia and sciatica were created by an imbalance of *apana vata*, which in turn was aggravating her *pitta*, giving rise to heart burn.

EXAMINING THE DHATUS

Next let us focus on the osteoarthritis, which is typical of a *vata* imbalance in the *asthi dhatu*, related also to the *apana vata* which in turn had pushed *vata* into the *majja dhatu*.

Physical examination begins with *rasa dhatu*. Here it can be concluded that the skin is indeed thin and there is a degree of dehydration and lack of nutrition. In cases like this, the anterior and inguinal lymph nodes should always be checked. They were not swollen in this particular case, but the blood vessels are sclerosed and there is evidence on taking the pulse of ventricular extra-systoles ('skipped' heart beats), indicating *prana* and *vyana vata* imbalances.

The *rakta dhatu* examination shows slightly raised blood pressure and *kapha* deposits in the coronary vessels, causing a blockage of *prana*. The *mamsa dhatu* seems minimally affected, as the nutrition, tone, power and coordination of the muscles appear to be in order. The accuracy of the *prana* and *vyana* vatas can be tested by asking Mrs R. to touch the nose with her index finger (*vyana*) and raising the leg from the knee (*apana*).

The *meda dhatu* is checked by seeing how much subcutaneous tissue there is present on the cheeks, breast, belly and bottom. In this particular case there is evidence of emaciation, illustrating a *vata* derangement. The *asthi dhatu* shows a poly-arthritis and there is reduced range of motion in all the joints. *Vata* is also deranged in the *majja dhatu*, causing the sciatica. Finally, the *shukra dhatu* is not relevant, as Mrs R. is post menopausal.

DIAGNOSIS
The conclusion of all of the foregoing diagnostic work is that Mrs R. has a type of dry asthma, due to *vata* aggravating *pitta* and literally drying everything out.

TREATMENT
The following herbs to be taken by mouth daily:
- yogamy guggalu
- ashwaghanda
- bala
- pippali
- abhrak bhasma.

- 1 cup of liquorice tea per day
- narayan oil to the chest and sciatic region, heated, before taking a bath
- oil enema once a week
- daily triphala
- yoga
- *pranayama* (breathing exercises)
- a *vata* pacifying diet.

OUTCOME

Mrs R. was experiencing less pain after six months, and her sleep had improved. She was able to reduce her prednisolone intake from 10 mg to 4 mg per day after one and a half years of treatment. All the treatments above help to pacify *vata* and improve the function of digestion and the alimentary canal.

CASE TWO
MISS D.

Miss D. is a graphic designer in her early thirties. Her hair is blond and fine and she has pale green eyes. Her skin is very pale and she appears run down. Her family history revealed an unhappy childhood, during which she felt emotionally deprived, her father eventually dying of alcohol abuse and aspirin consumption. She appeared immaculately presented, even though her self-esteem was very low.

MEDICAL HISTORY

Since she was twenty, Miss D. has had increasing pain in her joints, diagnosed by her GP as rheumatoid arthritis. Her condition appears to be exacerbated by consumption of potatoes, alcohol, cheese or suppression of emotions, as

well as cold weather or damp. Warmth seems to improve
the condition, which she best described as a 'burning
ache'. A skin rash appears in the winter months,
sometimes with small blisters. Congestion in the
lymphatics and sinuses cause a burning and stinging
sensation. She suffered glandular fever at the age of
twenty-two and has had sore throats from time to time
since she was eighteen.

THE EXAMINATION

Tongue examination revealed *ama* toxins in the colon and
there were ulcers present in the mouth. Her nails were
split and spoon shaped. Her *prakruti* was *vata* three, *pitta*
two, *kapha* one and her current constitution, or *vikruti*,
vata two, *pitta* three, *kapha* two (the numbers represent the
ratio of the three doshas to one another).

DIAGNOSIS

Vata from the colon had entered the joints. Dull aching in
the joints suggests *ama* toxins circulating in the system. *Vata*
has entered the *asthi dhatu*, leading to *ama vata* (rheumatoid
arthritis), triggered by all the factors listed in her history.
Pitta driven under the skin gives rise to the rash and there
is increased *pitta* in the liver. She is pale owing to anaemia.

TREATMENT

- herbs to pacify her *vata*
- triphala at night
- 1 cup ginger tea with 2 tsp castor oil to remove *ama*
- ginger and calamus root paste (1 tsp of each in a
  little water), for inflammation and pain
- ginger and baking soda baths (1 cup of each)
- a programme of meditation/yoga

OUTCOME

Miss D.'s pain was much reduced as long as she kept to the diet recommended. She had a greater range of motion in all her joints after twelve weeks of treatment.

CASE THREE
MISS C.

Miss C. was born in 1955 and works in a high profile, stressful job, which demands much travel and antisocial working hours. She is in the process of selling her house. As a baby, her frame was moderate, but Miss C.'s weight throughout her life has been more *kapha* in nature. Presently, her skin alternates between dryness and oiliness with acne occurring each month before her period. Her hair is soft, dark and oily, requiring frequent washing. Her appetite is good and she feels better when she avoids wheat, coffee and tea. Sometimes she feels slightly nauseous. She eats a lot of fruit and linseeds to help keep her bowel movements regular. Her father was domineering and aggressive and she feels that she has taken on some of his traits. (In ayurvedic medicine, the liver is associated with the emotion of anger, as it is in the west).

MEDICAL HISTORY

Miss C. complains of premenstrual tension, dysmenhorroea (painful periods) and increasing weight. She has phlegm in the back of her throat, lymphatic congestion in her breasts and intermittent constipation, which was her main concern. When stools do appear, they are thick, heavy and foul smelling, suggesting the presence of *ama*.

THE EXAMINATION

Examination of her tongue showed damp heat and toxins in the colon. She has brittle nails, which are thin and speckled. Poor liver and gall-bladder function (sclera and skin were slightly yellowish) were noted and she has passed numerous gall stones in the past. Her pulses showed a *pitta-kapha prakruti*, with a *vata* imbalance pushing the *pitta* higher.

TREATMENT

- liver flush, using 8 oz /200 g olive oil, 4 oz /100 g lime juice and garlic on rising (garlic causes dilation of the gall-bladder)
- no food till midday, for 3 days
- *vata* pacifying diet in the winter/spring
- *pitta* pacifying diet in the summer
- 1 tsp warm castor oil on the breasts; massage and then shower, daily
- tea for lymphatic congestion, after meals, made from: chamomile, basil, liquorice root
- practice yoga postures: camel, cobra, cow, spinal twists.

OUTCOME

Miss C. continues to lose weight — between 1-1½ lb/⅓–½ kg — a week. All the premenstrual symptoms improved immediately. The patient was having far less nausea after two weeks.

Sanskrit Glossary

Agni: fire, especially digestive fire

Alochak pitta: type of *pitta* related to vision

Ama: toxic material caused by poor digestion

Amla: sour taste

Ananda: bliss

Apana vata: 'downward' moving of the five breaths

Artha: goal of 'wealth'

Asana: yoga posture

Asthi: bone

Atman: inner self

Avalambak kapha: type of *Kapha* in the chest

Ayurveda: spiritual science of life

Bhakti yoga: yoga of devotion

Bhrajak pitta: type of *pitta* related to the complexion

Bhuta: element

Bodhak kapha: type of *kapha* giving rise to taste

Buddhi: 'organ' of discrimination

Chakra: spinal centre of energy

Charaka: author of old ayurvedic textbooks

Dharma: goal, ideal, law of one's nature

Dhatu: elemental tissue of the body

Dinacharya: daily regimen

Dosha: fault, primary force in body/mind

Doshic: quality relating to the doshas

Gunas: a principle quality of nature

Kapha: water/earth humor

Kledak kapha: type of *kapha* related to digestion

Mamsa: muscle

Manas: the concept of thought in the mind

Medas: fat tissue

Ojas: finest form of subtle energy/cement

Pachaka pitta: type of *pitta* related to digestion

Panchakarma: cleansing actions of vomiting, enemas, purgation, bleeding, and nasal medication

Pitta: biological fire/water humor

Prakruti: primary or basic constitution

Prana: breath of life

Pranayama: alternate nostril breathing exercises

Purusha: the inner self or person

Raga: desire

Rajas: *guna* principle of energy/activity/movement

Rajasic: having the quality of *rajas*

Rakta: blood

Ranjak pitta: type of *pitta* causing the colour of the blood

Rasa: a) plasma; b) taste

Sadhak pitta: type of *pitta* related to the brain

Samana vata: equalising breath

Samkhya: system of Indian philosophy (*sat* = 'truth'; *khya* = 'to know')

Sattva: *guna* of harmony and peace

Sattvic: having the quality of *sattva*

Shukra: reproductive fluids

Sleshak kapha: type of *kapha* lubricating the joints

Sukra: goal of happiness

Sushruta: author of old ayurvedic textbooks

Tamas: *guna* of inertia or mass

Tamasic: having the quality of *tamas*

Tanmantra: five principles of sense giving rise to the elements

Tarpak kapha: type of *kapha* related to the brain and nerves

Tejas: mental fire

Udana vata: 'upward' moving breath

Vayu: alternative name for *vata*

Vedas: ancient books of knowledge presenting the spiritual
    science of awareness

Vikruti: current state, or deviation from natural state of
    prakruti

Vyana vata: the outward moving of the five vatas or breaths

Appendix *Vata*

The diet should include:

*   40-50 % whole grain foods
*   10-20 % high quality protein
*   20-30 % fresh cooked vegetables
*   10 % or more of fresh fruit

— *OK very occasionally* ★ — *OK in moderation only*

FRUITS

No Dried fruit; Apples (raw); Cranberries; Pears;
Persimmon; Pomegranate; Prunes (soaked); Quince;
Watermelon.

Note : *Fruits and fruit juices are best consumed by themselves for all doshas.*

Yes Applesauce; Sweet fruits; Apricots; Avocado;
Bananas; All berries; Cherries; Coconut; Dates;
Fresh figs; Grapefruit; Grapes; Kiwi; Lemons; Limes;
Mango; Nectarines; Oranges; Papaya; Peaches;
Pineapples; Plums; Rhubarb; Soursop; Strawberries;
Sweet melons.

VEGETABLES

No *In general, dried, frozen or raw vegetables;* Aubergine
(eggplant); Beet greens; Broccoli; Burdock root;
Cabbage; Cauliflower; Celery; Fresh corn; Jerusalem
artichoke; Jicama; Kale; Kohlrabi; Leafy greens;
Lettuce; Mushrooms (raw); Onions (raw); Parsley;
Peas (raw); Peppers; Potato (white); Spaghetti squash;
Spinach (raw); Sprouts (all); Tomatoes (raw);
Turnips; Turnip greens.

Yes *In general, most cooked vegetables;* Acorn squash;
Artichoke; Asparagus; Beets; Butternut squash;
Carrots; Cilantro; Courgette (zucchini); Cucumber;
Daikon radish; Fenugreek greens; Green beans (well
cooked); Horseradish; Leeks (cooked); Mustard
greens; Okra (cooked); Olives (black and green);
Onion (cooked); Parsnip; Potato (sweet); Pumpkin;
Radish; Swede (rutabaga); Scallopini squash; Spinach
(cooked); Summer squash; Tomato (cooked);
Watercress; Winter squash.

GRAINS

No Barley; Bread (yeast); Buckwheat; Cold, dry, puffed
cereals; Corn; Granola; Millet; Oats (dry); Oat bran;
Rice cakes; Rye; Sago; Wheat bran.

Yes Amaranth*; Oats (cooked); Quinoa; Rice (all
varieties); Sprouted wheat bread; Wheat.

ANIMAL FOODS

No Lamb; Pork; Rabbit; Venison.

Yes Beef; Buffalo; Chicken; Duck; Eggs (including duck
eggs); Fish; Seafood; Shrimp; Turkey.

LEGUMES

No Aduki beans; Black beans; Black-eyed peas; Brown
lentils; Chick peas (garbanzos); Dried peas; Kidney
beans; Lima beans; Navy beans; Pinto beans; Soy
beans; Soy flour; Soy powder; Spilt peas; Tempeh;
Tofu#; White beans.

Yes Black lentils; Miso*; Mung beans; Mung dal; Red
lentils*; Soy cheese*; Soy milk (liquid)*; Soy sauce*;
Tepery beans; Tofu; Tur dal.

NUTS

No *None listed.*

Yes Almonds; Black walnuts; Brazil nuts; Cashews;
Coconut; English walnuts; Filberts; Hazelnuts;
Macadamia nuts; Peanuts*; Pecans; Pine nuts;
Pistachios; Walnuts.

SEEDS

No Psyllium#; Popcorn.

Yes Chia; Flax; Pumpkin; Sesame; Sunflower.

CONDIMENTS

No Chilli pepper#; Ginger (dry); Ketchup#; Onion (raw).

Yes Black pepper*; Black sesame seeds; Chutney;
Coconut; Coriander leaves*; Cottage cheese;
Grated cheese; Daikon radish; Dulse; Fresh ginger;
Garlic; Ghee; Gomasio; Hijiki; Horseradish;
Kelp; Kombu; Lemon; Lime; Mango chutney;
Mayonnaise; Mint leaves; Mustard; Onion (cooked);
Papaya chutney; Pickles; Salt; Seaweed (wet).

SWEETENERS

No White sugar; Maple syrup#.

Yes Barley malt syrup; Brown rice syrup; Fructose; Fruit
juice (concentrated); Honey; Jaggary; Molasses;
Natural sugar*; Sucanat; Sugar cane juice.

DAIRY

No Cow's milk (powder); Goat's milk (powder); Hard
cheese#; Yoghurt.

Yes *All OK in moderation:* Butter; Buttermilk; Cow's
milk; Cottage cheese; Goat's milk; Goat's cheese; Ice
cream*; Soft cheese; Sour cream*.

OILS

No Flax seed.

Yes *All oils OK, especially:* Olive; Sesame. *External use only:* Coconut.

SPICES

No Caraway.

Yes Ajwan; Allspice; Almond extract; Amchoor; Anise; Asafoetida; Basil; Bay leaf; Black pepper; Cardamom; Cayenne★; Cloves; Coriander; Cumin; Dill; Fennel; Fenugreek★; Garlic; Ginger; Horseradish; Mace; Marjoram; Mint; Mustard seeds; Nutmeg; Onion (cooked); Orange peel; Oregano; Paprika; Parsley; Peppermint; Pippali; Poppy seeds; Rosemary; Rose water; Saffron; Sage; Savory; Spearmint; Star anise; Tamarind; Tarragon; Thyme; Turmeric; Vanilla; Wintergreen.

BEVERAGES

No Apple juice; Carob#; Carbonated drinks; Chocolate; Coffee; Cold milk drinks; Cranberry juice; Fig shake; Ice cold drinks; Pear juice; Pungent teas; Prune juice#; Tea (black); Tomato juice; V-8 juice; **Herb teas:** Alfalfa#; Barley#; Blackberry; Borage#; Burdock; Chrysanthemum#; Cornsilk; Dandelion; Ginseng; Hibiscus; Hops#; Hyssop#; Jasmine#; Mormon tea; Nettle#; Passion flower#; Red clover#; Red zinger; Sage; Strawberry#; Violet#; Wintergreen#; Yarrow; Yerba mate#.

Yes Alcohol★; Almond drink; Aloe vera juice; Apricot juice; Banana shake; Berry juice; Carrot juice; Carrot/ginger juice; Cherry juice; Cider; Coconut milk; Hot dairy drinks; Grape juice; Grapefruit

juice; Lemonade; Mango juice; Miso broth; Mixed
vegetable juice; Hot spiced milk; Orange juice;
Papaya juice; Peach nectar; Pineapple juice; Sour
juices and teas; Soy milk (well spiced and hot);
Grain teas: Cafix; Roma; Pero; **Herb teas:** Ajwan;
Bansha (with milk sweetener); Basil*; Catnip*;
Chamomile; Cinnamon*; Clove; Comfrey;
Elderflower; Eucalyptus; Fennel; Fenugreek; Ginger
(fresh); Hawthorn; Juniper berry; Lavender; Lemon
balm; Lemon grass; Licorice; Lotus; Marshmallow;
Oat straw; Orange peel; Osha; Pennyroyal;
Peppermint; Raspberry*; Rose flower; Rose hip;
Saffron; Sarsaparilla; Sassafras; Spearmint; Wild
ginger.

OTHER
No *None listed.*
Yes Spirulina and other blue-green algae.

Appendix *Pitta*

The diet should include:

*   40-50 % whole grain foods
*   15-20 % high quality protein
*   30-40 % fresh cooked vegetables
*   15 % or more of fresh fruit

— *OK very occasionally* ★ — *OK in moderation only*

FRUITS

No   *When any of the following are sour they should not be eaten;* Apples; Apricots; Bananas; Berries; Cherries; Cranberries; Grapefruit; Green grapes; Kiwi#; Lemons; Oranges; Papaya#; Peaches; Pineapples; Persimmon; Plums; Rhubarb; Soursop; Strawberries; Tamarind.

Yes   *When the following are sweet they are OK to eat;* Apples; Apricots; Avocado; Berries; Cherries; Coconut; Dates; Figs; Limes★; Mango; Melons; Oranges; Pineapples; Plums; Pears; Pomegranate; Prunes; Quince; Raisins; Red grapes; Watermelon.

VEGETABLES

No   Aubergine (eggplant)#; Beet greens; Beets (raw); Carrots (raw); Daikon radish; Fresh corn; Fenugreek greens; Garlic; Green olives; Horseradish; Kohlrabi#; Leeks (raw); Mustard greens; Onions (raw); Peppers (hot); Radish; Spinach (raw); Tomatoes; Turnips; Turnip greens.

Yes   Acorn squash; Artichoke; Asparagus; Beets (cooked); Broccoli; Brussels sprouts; Burdock root; Butternut

squash; Cabbage; Capsicum (bell pepper); Carrots
(cooked); Cauliflower; Courgette (zucchini);
Cucumber; Celery; Cilantro; Fennel; Green beans;
Green peppers; Jerusalem artichoke; Jicama; Kale;
Leafy greens; Leeks (cooked); Lettuce; Mushrooms;
Okra; Olives (black); Onions (cooked); Parsley;
Parsnip; Peas; Pumpkin (cooked); Swede (rutabaga);
Scallopini squash; Spaghetti squash; Spinach
(cooked); Summer squash; Sweet potatoes;
Watercress★; White potatoes; Winter squash.

GRAINS

No   Buckwheat; Corn; Millet; Oats (dry); Oat granola;
      Quinoa; Rice (brown)#; Rye.

Yes   Amaranth; Barley; Couscous; Oat bran★; Oats
      (cooked); Rice (basmati); Rice cakes; Rice (white);
      Wheat; Wheat bran; Wheat granola.

ANIMAL FOOD

No   Beef; Duck; Egg yolk; Lamb; Pork; Salmon; Seafood.

Yes   Buffalo; Egg white; Freshwater fish (including
      shrimp★); Rabbit; Venison; White chicken;
      White turkey.

LEGUMES

No   Black lentils; Tur dal; Urad dal.

Yes   Aduki beans; Black beans; Black-eyed peas; Chana
      dal; Chick peas (garbanzos); Kidney beans; Lentils
      (red and brown); Lima beans; Mung beans; Navy
      beans; Pinto beans; Soy beans; Soy products: Soy
      cheese; Soy flour★; Soy milk (liquid); Soy powder★;
      Split peas; Tempeh; Tepery beans; Tofu; White
      beans.

NUTS

No Almonds (plus skin); Black walnuts; Brazil nuts;
Cashews; English walnuts; Filberts; Hazelnuts;
Macadamia nuts; Peanuts; Pecans; Pine nuts;
Pistachios.

Yes Almonds (soaked and peeled); Coconut.

SEEDS

No Chia; Sesame.

Yes Flax; Psyllium; Pumpkin*; Sunflower.

CONDIMENTS

No Black sesame seeds; Chilli peppers; Daikon radish;
Garlic; Ginger; Gomasio; Grated cheese;
Horseradish; Kelp; Ketchup; Mustard; Lemon;
Lime; Lime pickle; Mango pickle; Mayonnaise;
Onion (raw); Papaya chutney; Pickles; Radish;
Salt#; Seaweed (unrinsed)#; Sesame seeds; Soy sauce;
Tamarind#; Yogurt (undiluted).

Yes Black pepper*; Coconut; Coriander leaves; Cottage
cheese; Dulse (well-rinsed)*; Ghee; Hijiki (well-
rinsed)*; Kombu*; Lettuce; Mango chutney;
Mint leaves.

SWEETENERS

No Honey; Jaggery; Molasses.

Yes Barley malt syrup; Brown rice syrup; Fruit juice
(concentrate); Fructose; Maple syrup; Natural sugar;
Sucanat; Sugar cane juice; White sugar*.

DAIRY

No Buttermilk; Feta cheese; Hard cheese; Salted butter;
Sour cream; Yogurt.

Yes Cottage cheese; Dilute yogurt (1:2-3 pts water);
Mild soft cheese; Ghee; Cow's milk; Goat's milk; Ice
cream; Unsalted butter.

OILS

No Almond; Apricot; Corn; Safflower; Sesame.

Yes *In moderation :* Flax seed; Olive; Sunflower; Sesame;
Soy; Walnut.

SPICES

No Ajwan; Allspice; Almond extract; Amchoor; Anise;
Asafoetida; Basil; Bay leaf; Caraway#; Cayenne;
Cloves; Dry ginger; Fenugreek; Garlic (raw);
Horseradish; Mace; Marjoram; Mustard seeds;
Nutmeg; Onion (raw); Oregano; Paprika; Pippali;
Poppy seeds; Rosemary; Sage; Savory; Star anise;
Tamarind; Tarragon; Thyme.

Yes Basil leaves; Black pepper*; Cardamom*;
Cinnamon; Coriander; Cumin; Dill; Fennel; Fresh
ginger; Mint; Neem leaves*; Orange peel*; Parsley*;
Peppermint; Rose water; Saffron; Spearmint;
Turmeric; Vanilla*; Wintergreen.

BEVERAGES

No Alcohol (spirits/wine); Banana shake; Berry juice
(sour); Carbonated drinks; Cherry juice (sour);
Coffee; Carrot juice; Carrot/ginger juice;
Carrot/vegetable; Chocolate; Cranberry juice;
Grapefruit; Highly salted drinks; Ice cold drinks;
Lemonade; Orange juice#; Miso broth#; Papaya
juice; Pineapple juice; Pungent teas; Sour juices
and teas; Tomato juice; V-8 Juice; **Herb teas:**
Ajwan; Basil#; Cinnamon#; Cloves; Dry ginger;

Eucalyptus; Fenugreek; Ginseng; Hawthorn; Hyssop; Juniper berry; Mormon tea; Osha; Pennyroyal; Red zinger; Rosehip; Sage; Sassafras; Wild ginger; Yerba mate.

Yes Alcohol (beer)*; Almond drink; Aloe vera juice; Apple juice; Apricot juice; Berry juice (sweet); Carob; Cherry juice (sweet); Coconut milk; Cool dairy drinks; Date shake; Fig shake; Goat's milk; Grape juice; Mango juice; Mixed vegetable juice; Peach nectar; Pear juice; Pomegranate juice; Prune juice; Soy milk; Vegetable bouillon; **Grain teas:** Cafix; Roma; Pero; **Herb teas:** Alfalfa; Bansha; Blackberry; Barley; Borage; Burdock; Catnip; Chamomile; Chicory; Chrysanthemum; Comfrey; Cornsilk; Dandelion; Elder flower; Fennel; Fresh ginger; Hibiscus; Hops; Jasmine; Lavender; Lemon balm; Lemon grass; Licorice; Lotus; Marshmallow; Nettle; Oat straw; Orange peel*; Passion flower; Peppermint; Raspberry; Red clover; Rose flower; Saffron; Sarsaparilla; Spearmint; Strawberry; Violet; Wintergreen; Yarrow.

OTHER

No Spirulina and other blue-green algae.

Yes *None listed.*

Appendix *Kapha*

The diet should include:

- 30–40 % whole grain foods
- 20 % high quality protein
- 40–50 % fresh cooked vegetables
- 10 % or more of fresh fruit

— *OK very occasionally* ★ — *OK in moderation only*

FRUITS

No Avocado; Bananas: Coconut; Dates; Fresh figs; Grapefruit; Grapes#; Kiwi; Lemons#: Limes#; Mangoes#; Melons; Oranges; Papaya; Pineapples; Plums; Rhubarb; Soursop; Tamarind; Watermelon.

Yes Apples: Apple sauce; Apricots; Berries; Cherries; Cranberries; Dry figs★; Peaches; Pears; Persimmon; Pomegranate; Prunes; Quince; Raisins; Strawberries★.

VEGETABLES

No Acorn squash; Butternut squash; Courgette (zucchini); Cucumber; Olives; Parsnip#; Pumpkin; Raw tomatoes; Spaghetti squash#; Sweet potatoes; Taro root; Winter squash.

Yes *Steamed, raw, pungent and bitter vegetables;* Artichoke; Asparagus; Aubergine (eggplant); Beets; Beet Greens; Capsicum (bell pepper); Broccoli; Brussels sprouts; Burdock root; Cabbage; Carrots; Cauliflower; Celery; Daikon radish; Dandelion greens; Fennel; Fenugreek greens; Garlic; Green beans; Green chillies; Horseradish; Jerusalem

artichoke; Jicama; Kale; Kohlrabi; Leaf greens (kale);
Leeks; Lettuce; Mushrooms; Mustard greens; Okra;
Onions; Parsley; Peas; Radish; Scallopini squash;
Spinach; Summer squash; Swede (rutabaga);
Sweetcorn; Sweet, hot peppers; Turnips; Turnip
greens; Yel crickneck squash; Watercress; White
potatoes.

GRAINS

No   Brown rice; Oats (cooked); Quinoa#; Rice cakes#;
Spelt#; Wheat; White rice.

Yes   Amaranth*; Barley; Basmati rice (with clove or
peppercorns)*; Buckwheat; Corn; Couscous;
Granola (low-fat); MilletOats (dry); Oat bran;
Polenta; Rye; Wheat bran; Sago; Sprouted wheat
bread (essene); Tapioca.

ANIMAL FOODS

No   Beef; Buffalo; Duck; Lamb; Pork; Salmon; Sea fish;
Seafood; Tuna.

Yes   ChickenEggs (not fried or scrambled with fat);
Freshwater fish; Turkey; Rabbit; Shrimp; Venison.

LEGUMES

No   Black lentils; Cold tofu; Common lentils; Soy beans;
Cold soy milk; Kidney beans; Mung beans#; Soy
cheese; Soy flour; Soy powder; Tempeh.

Yes   Aduki beans; Black beans; Black-eyed peas; Chana
dal; Chick peas (garbanzos); Hot tofu*; Kala chana;
Lima beans; Navy beans; Pinto beans; Red/brown
lentils; Soy milk; Soy sausages; Split peas; Tempeh;
Tepery beans; Tur dal; White beans.

NUTS

No Almond (soaked/peeled)#; Black walnuts; Brazil nuts; Cashews; Coconut; English walnut; Filberts; Hazelnuts; Macadamia nuts; Peanuts; Pecans; Pine nuts; Pistachios.

Yes *None listed.*

SEEDS

No Psyllium#; Sesame.

Yes Chia; Flax★; Popcorn (no salt, no butter); Pumpkin★; Sunflower★.

CONDIMENTS

No Black sesame seeds; Cottage cheese; Grated cheese; Hijiki#; Kelp; Ketchup#; Kombu; Lemon#; Lime; Lime pickle; Mango chutney; Mango pickles; Mayonnaise; Papaya chutney; Pickles; Salt; Seaweed (well-rinsed)#; Sesame seeds; Soy sauce; Tamarind; Vinegar: Yogurt.

Yes Black pepper; Chili pepper; Coriander leaves; Daikon radish; Dry ginger; Dulse (well-rinsed)★; Garlic; Ghee; Horseradish; Lettuce; Mint leaves; Mustard; Onions; Radish.

SWEETENERS

No Barley malt syrup; Brown rice syrup; Fructose; Jaggery; Maple syrup; Molasses; Natural sugar; Sucanat; Sugar cane juice; White sugar.

Yes Raw honey★; Fruit juice (concentrate).

DAIRY

No Butter (salted); Butter (unsalted)#; Buttermilk; Cheese of all kinds; Cows milk; Ice cream; Sour cream; Yogurt (undiluted).

Yes Cottage cheese (from skimmed goat's milk); Ghee★;
Goat's milk; Dilute yogurt (1:4 pts water); Goat's
cheese (not aged and unsalted).

OILS

No Avocado; Apricot; Coconut; Flax seed#; Olive;
Primrose; Safflower; Sesame (internally); Soy;
Walnut.

Yes Almond★; Corn★; Sunflower★.

SPICES

No *None listed.*

Yes Ajwan; Allspice; Almond extract; Anise; Asafoetida;
Basil; Bay leaf; Black pepper; Caraway; Cardamom;
Cayenne; Cinnamon; Cloves; Coriander; Cumin;
Dill; Dry ginger; Fennel★; Fenugreek; Garlic;
Horseradish; Mace; Mango chutney; Marjoram;
Mint; Mustard seeds; Neem leaves; Nutmeg; Onion;
Orange peel; Oregano; Paprika; Parsley;
Peppermint; Pippali; Poppy seeds; Rosemary; Rose
water; Saffron; Sage; Savory; Spearmint; Sprouts;
Star anise; Tarragon; Thyme; Turmeric; Vanilla★;
Wintergreen.

BEVERAGES

No Alcohol (beer, spirits and sweet wines); Almond
drink; Banana shake; Carbonated drinks; Cold dairy
drinks; Coconut milk; Coffee#; Chocolate; Date
shake; Grapefruit juice; Highly salted drinks; Ice
cold drinks; Lemonade; Miso broth; Orange juice;
Papaya juice; Pineapple juice#; Rice milk; Sour
juices and teas; Soy milk (cold); Tomato juice; V-8
juice; **Herb teas:** Comfrey; Lotus; Marshmallow;
Oat straw; Red zinger; Rosehip#.

Yes Alcohol, dry (red or white); Aloe vera juice; Apple
juice*; Apricot juice; Berry juice; Black tea; Carob;
Carrot juice; Carrot-ginger juice; Carrot juice
combinations; Cherry juice (sweet); Cranberry juice;
Fig shake; Hot spiced goat's milk*; Grape juice;
Mango juice; Mixed vegetable juice; Peach nectar;
Pear juice; Pomegranate juice; Pungent teas; Prune
juice; Soy milk (well-spiced and warm); **Grain teas:**
Cafix; **Herb teas:** Ajwan; Alfalfa; Barley; Basil;
Bansha; Blackberry; Borage; Burdock; Catnip;
Chamomile; Chicory; Chrysanthemum; Cinnamon;
Cloves; Corn; Silk; Dandelion; Dry ginger; Elder
flower; Eucalyptus; Fennel*; Fenugreek; Ginseng*;
Hawthorn; Hibiscus; Hops; Hyssop; Jasmine; Juniper
berries; Lavender; Lemon balm; Lemon grass;
Licorice*; Mormon tea; Nettle; Orange peel; Osha;
Passion flower; Pennyroyal; Peppermint; Raspberry;
Red clover; Rose flower; Saffron; Sage;
Sarsaparilla*; Sassafras; Spearmint; Strawberry;
Violet; Wild ginger; Wintergreen; Yarrow; Yerba
mate.

OTHER

No Potassium salts.

Yes Brewer's yeast; Spirulina and other blue-green algae.

Herbs and Spices to Assist in Balancing the Doshas

B elow is a table of common herbs and spices used in cooking, and their properties in terms of their effect upon *vata*, *pitta* and *kapha*. Use them to modify the effects of the foods you are preparing in the direction indicated in the table.

'+' indicates that it aggravates the *dosha*

'–' indicates that it reduces or pacifies the *dosha*

'~' indicates no effect one way or the other

Herb/spice	*Vata*	*Pitta*	*Kapha*
Alfalfa	–	~	–
Aloe Vera	–	–	–
Cardamom	–	+ (in excess)	–
Cayenne pepper	–	+	–
Cinnamon	–	– (small amounts)	–
Cloves	–	+	–
Coriander	–	–	–
Cumin	~	–	–
Garlic	–	+	–
Ghee	–	–	–
Ginger	–	+	–
Honey (uncooked)	–	~	–
Licorice	~	–	~
Mustard	–	+	–
Nutmeg	–	– (small amounts)	–
Pepper	–	+	–
Salt	~	+	+
Turmeric	– (small amounts)	– (small amounts)	–

Helpful Addresses

Australia

The Australian School of Ayurveda
27 Blight Street, Ridleyton, South Australia 5008.

United Kingdom

Ayurvedic Living
P O Box 188, Exeter EX4 5AB.

The Yoga for Health Foundation
Ickwell Bury, Biggleswade, Bedfordshire SG18 9EF.

United States

American Holistic Medical Association
4101 Lake Boone Trail, Suite 201, Raleigh,
North Carolina 27607.

The Ayurvedic Institute
P O Box 23445, Albuquerque, New Mexico 87192-1445.

Recommended Reading

Bhagwan Dash, Vaidya, *A Handbook of Ayurveda*,
New Delhi, India: 1983.

Frawley, David, *Ayurvedic Healing: A Comprehensive Guide*,
Salt Lake City, USA: Passage Press 1992.

Heyn, Birgit, *Ayurvedic Medicine: The Gentle Strength of
Indian Healing*, Wellingborough: Thorsons 1987.

Lad, Vasant, *Ayurveda: The Science of Self-Healing*,
Sante Fe, USA: Lotus Press 1984.

Lad, Vasant and Frawley, David, *The Yoga of Herbs,*
Sante Fe, USA: Lotus Press 1986.

Lad, Usha and Lad, Vasant, *Ayurvedic Cooking for Self-
Healing*, Albuquerque, USA: The Ayurvedic Press 1994.

Murthy, K. R. Sikantha (tr.), *Astanga Hrdayam*
(Vols. 1, 2 and 3), Varanasi, India: 1992.

Ranade, Subhash, *Natural Healing Through Ayurveda*,
Salt Lake City, USA: Passage Press 1993.

Svoboda, Robert, *Ayurveda: Life, Health and Longevity*,
London: Arkana 1992

Svoboda, Robert, *Prakruti: Your Ayurvedic Constitution*,
Albuquerque, USA: Geocom 1988.

Index